Autism in Kids

Parent's Guide to Autism Treatment and Support

(Using Daily Activities to Help Kids Communicate Learn and Connect)

Melissa Werner

Published By **Chris David**

Melissa Werner

All Rights Reserved

Autism in Kids: Parent's Guide to Autism Treatment and Support (Using Daily Activities to Help Kids Communicate Learn and Connect)

ISBN 978-1-77485-740-3

No part of this guidebook shall be reproduced in any form without permission in writing from the publisher except in the case of brief quotations embodied in critical articles or reviews.

Legal & Disclaimer

The information contained in this ebook is not designed to replace or take the place of any form of medicine or professional medical advice. The information in this ebook has been provided for educational & entertainment purposes only.

The information contained in this book has been compiled from sources deemed reliable, and it is accurate to the best of the Author's knowledge; however, the Author cannot guarantee its accuracy and validity and cannot be held liable for any errors or omissions. Changes are periodically made to this book. You must consult your doctor or get professional medical advice before using any of the suggested remedies, techniques, or information in this book.

TABLE OF CONTENTS

Introduction

In the 21st century we have access to many sources of information, but we have a limited understanding of. Everything you want to know is just a mouse click away, yet millions of people make judgments and provide bad advice on autism. The book we'll examine the subject in depth and examine the parenting of autistic children from a variety of different perspectives. Parenting is hard enough already and receiving bad guidance only increases the burden. As we explore the subject broadly, we'll look at the causes and examine certain aspects of what this book covers and doesn't.

Chapter 1: Toddler Parenting Overview

Being a parentis a wonderful experience. Anyone can determine what's going on in your head. You feel such affection for your child, that you're often afraid your chest is about to burst. You are also always concerned about the safety of your child. You're trying to ensure that they're safe throughout the day. It is possible that you would think you can have control over everything they do. These feelings are not uncommon and are an expected aspect of parenting.

It's possible that what's not apparent to you is what's going inside the brain of your child. For adults, you could simply inquire about what they're thinking and, eventually they'll share their thoughts with you. However, understanding what's happening in the mind of a toddler is more challenging. The brains of toddlers operate in a different way than yours. They are still in the process of developing and they're trying to comprehend the world around them. Additionally, since they're relatively new in the field, they are able to conceptualize things by themselves, from what they've learned, which isn't very much. When you combine these two factors, you'll have a thinking process that's completely different from what you possess. Unfortunately, you don't understand their thinking. Or , can you?

The brain development of your child

"Why do you bite me with no motive?" "Why would you decide to put it into the mouth of someone else?" "It's just water. Why would you be scared to drink drinking water?" Do these questions are familiar? If yes likely because you're always considering about your child. Before you can solve these issues, it's important to understand the fundamentals of how the brain of your toddler operates.

One reason you are unable to understand why your child performs the actions you see him doing is because his reasoning process is still in development He isn't certain if he comprehends why he is doing the things that he does. It is crucial that you know what your child is thinking about and trying to instill into his own. These early years will decide who your child grows to be and you must influence as much as you possibly can.

The following picture will give you an overall understanding of the development your child is experiencing. Between the ages of 1 and 2 toddlers learn through sensory input. They also experience and perceive objects. Their goal at this point is to develop the ability to react to their environment. As they age they also experience emotions and experiences like eating and rocking. They rely on their caregivers to offer not only physical assistance, but also emotional support too. Their need for emotional assistance is heightened when they're stressed.

From 2 to 7 will observe your child attempting to cultivate imagination and creativity. They will also learn the ability to think such as reasoning, memory, logic emotional awareness, attention, and attention. These changes make this stage of life extremely important. When your toddler's memory starts to develop, will be able to recall things more clearly. Additionally, he will be able to process symbols and comprehend abstract concepts. At this point, your child may also be able to consider the past and future in a certain degree.

As all of these changes are happening the mind of your toddler is also susceptible to being influenced by external influences. In reality, all of these changes are due to some influence from outside. To simplify things we can reduce it down to three categories which are: biological factors, environmental factors, and interpersonal interactions.

The environmental aspects comprise things like diet and nutrition as well as space for exploration, the ability to learn and have access to reading as well as relationships with family members. When we talk about biological aspects, we're referring to issues like social and family treatment as well as how healthy the children as well as familymembers, and, most importantly, the child's sexual. Girls and boys differ from one another. The influence of interpersonal relationships on the development of a child includes aspects like the attachment to the caregivers and parents, as well as the social circle of friends, and , of course, the parenting style.

It's impossible to control these elements. Some would consider you crazy if you tried. Understanding the roles of each can assist you in adjusting the way you interact to and interact with your child.

What are the reasons they behave as they do?

As an adult, you are aware more than any other person that toddlers need to be cared for. It is how long you've been in your relationship with the child from when the time he was born has given you any knowledge. The reason they make the choices they do is pretty straightforward. They are doing what they have to do. Similar to it being illogical to inquire about what toddlers do when they eat or sleep and sleep, it's just as unlogical to ask them why they have temper tantrums. In the end, parents are thankful for the things their children can do without instructions or demands. For instance, breathing for instance. However, you need to remind them of other activities, such as feeding and sleeping. However, the fact remains that toddlers can do things on their own which is a great thing.

In the case of psychological behaviors, such as emotions and choices, children do not need to be trained. Think about the following patterns such as. The desire for survival as well as belonging and love as well as freedom, power and, of course, affection. It is not necessary to encourage your child to have these desires. While there are more emotional and psychological traits than those five, they're fundamental, and form the basis for everything else. If you study them carefully you can see the areas of intersection between your actions and those of others. These are the places where your actions and motives behind them are in line with the behavior of your children. Therefore, when you are trying to comprehend your child's behavior you must keep these behaviors in your thoughts.

Take a look at crying for instance. Why do toddlers cry? That's quite simple, right? They cry because they're angry, hungry or tired, unhappy, hungry, or cranky or simply are bored or stop playing. There are a myriad of reasons that toddlers cry. Analyzing the environment of a toddler can provide a accurate idea of what they are feeling and what they would like. However, the amount of understanding you gain will differ based on a variety of factors, such as those mentioned earlier under the heading of developmental factors. But, having a basic understanding that there are these variables can improve your understanding of the reasons behind the things they do.

To delve a bit deeper to understand the behavior of your child look at the four different levels of behaviour for children. The actions are deliberate, effective, responsible, or consistent with established guidelines. Therefore, if your child is crying for a lollipop it is a deliberate act. However, is it successful? It will be determined by whether or your role being a responsible parent accept the request. What is appropriate or not? There are many methods to evaluate this act in accordance with the rules you've set within your home. However, the most common idea is this. When the lollipops belong somebody else then the actions are absolutely not liable. The accountability of the act is also closely linked to the connection to established laws and regulations.

When all is done and dusted as you parent, it's essential to recognize that, even though your toddler's actions might not be in line with all these boxes, your toddler is doing what is best for him/her to do to the best of their capability. Many times, toddlers who aren't careful do not realize they're in fact naughty. They have to be taught.

Helping toddlers flourish

If you've been a parent previously, chances are that you're familiar with at most of the procedures within this article. Your primary responsibility as an adult is to establish the right environment for your children so that they have the autonomy and understanding to develop and express themselves effectively. A lot of parents feel that the process of preparing their child for life in general is more of an introspective effort. It's not like you wake up every day and think that to yourself "I'm trying to ensure that my child will excel regardless of the path it requires." It's more likely to think of that "I wish for my son to attend a top school and be able to get top grades." However at the core of all that is that you desire your child to live a an amazing life. This is flourishing.

We'll cover plenty of advice and tips on creating a healthy and happy atmosphere for the toddlers in your home in the upcoming chapters. While we're here, let's look at three simple methods to encourage an appropriate development for your child.

In the first place, you shouldn't inform them that they can be anything they choose to be. This might seem like an odd advice, but it's supported by research. The research conducted in the name of the market research company, C+R research, found that the younger generation particularly Americans aren't looking for jobs that are designed toward the future. People are much more fascinated by athletics, music as well as video gaming. Informing your children that they could be anything they'd like to become could end up leading them to a life of unemployed. It's better to advise that they focus on prospective jobs in fields like construction and healthcare.

Secondly, don't skip eating dinner together. Many parents prefer to eat dinner with their children, but at the point at which bills and other obligations make them take progressively larger portions of their family time. The suggestion to always have dinner with your family is supported through research carried out by a non-profit group which is based at Harvard University. The study found that children who eat dinner with their families for at most five days each week had lower risk of using substances as compared to other children. Additionally, they have better GPAs, better confidence in themselves and a better vocabulary. The connection isn't understood yet but it's obvious.

Finally, you must enforce the concept of a "no-screen" time limit for your children. We'll go deeper about the necessity of schedules in the chapter. For this moment, let's look at the negative impact of screens that are plugged into the children's brains. Research has shown that screens for technology can trigger permanent brain changes of children. The term in this case is modification and not injury. According to the American Academy of Pediatrics recommends that children younger than 18 months old shouldn't be exposed to screens in any way, aside from video chat. It's not possible to deprive them of the time they spend with dad or mommy.

Self-Regulation and the Strategies for Success

The ability to regulate emotions is something that parents want in their child. Imagine if your child knew when to throw a temper tantrum and when to be a good boy. If your child knew when to chew an lollipop, and when to let it alone, then parenting will be a total pleasure. Since that's not happened so far, you can be sure that it will never happen, not alone anyway. You have a significant role to play in ensuring your children know what to do.

In order to approach self-regulation, Scott Bezsylko, the director of the Winston Prep Schools for children with learning difficulties, has an important point to remember. He suggests that self-regulation be approached the same manner as other abilities in the life of a toddler are taken care of. Skills such as academic excellence and social wellbeing. According to his research, thinking of emotional self-regulation as something that can be taught alters how you view it, as well as the way your child perceives it. It is important to help them learn how to deal with difficult situations with the necessary scaffolding. It is basically introducing them to it , one step at each step.

For a final instance you can think about solving difficult math homework. The most effective method to tackle it is to create the foundation, which is by solving one issue for your child, and then allowing your child to tackle the other problems. It is important to allow the child to test his skills to make mistakes. As time passes, keep making progress and you'll see the child's skills increase.

We are now at the conclusion of this chapter. Through this section, you must be able to recognize that the brain of your toddler is a bit different than yours. You'll be able to recognize that, despite the distinction in behavior however, the same motivations are driving each of you. The most basic motivation is the desire to survive. As the activities get more complex and the motivations become more complex, so too do the actions. But, they're all built on the same structure. You must also know how to help your child's future success by implementing evidence-based guidelines, such as limiting screen time, a deliberate career guidance, and eating dinner together as the family. In the final part, we talked about ways you can develop emotional self-regulation in your children.

These are mainly geared to parenting children who don't possess Autism Spectrum Disorder. In the next chapters we'll give the condition the full attention it deserves and provide an easy-to-follow guide to parenting children with ASD.

Chapter 2: Social Interaction For Children With Autism

The most significant issues that children who have autism encounter is engaging in social interactions, as well as maintaining relationships. They aren't able to respond to and process information in the manner one would imagine. Autism-related children often experience new experiences that make them uncomfortable, which is why it's essential to be aware of the issues they face and teach them how to manage potentially stressful situations.

Social skills are essential for everyone, as they are essential for survival, and each human being requires these skills to thrive and function. Particularly in the modern world. Social skills help you build and sustain relationships as well as participate in exercises for building community. They are also directly tied to feelings of emotional satisfaction, such as joy and affection. Learning to teach your child social skills will allow him to build friendships as well as maintain relationships and enable him to become productive social members.

Unfortunately, mastering social abilities and cues is somewhat more difficult for those who have autism. They struggle to comprehend the social norms and rules that guide our interactions with others. Therefore, they often require explicit instructions and lots of time to integrate fully. Individuals with ASD typically seek to overcome this by trying to understand what society is like for them. Most of the time the attempts they make at social interaction are perceived as being unnatural and could even cause harm and offence to people. As their guardians, mentors and parents, it is your responsibility to take care of your children by teaching them the proper social skills and rules that they should follow in order to fit into society in their own way.

Social skills teaching

Children who suffer from ASD differ greatly from one another and it's impossible to follow a single strategy or approach when trying in teaching your child something important as social abilities. Before you begin in teaching them the skills you believe is the right social skills, you need to know what areas your child is struggling with.

There are four issues that children with ASD generally face. They are unable to express their feelings or think to people, and they're sometimes unaware of certain rules. They can also be troubled communicating through non-verbal cues in addition to starting as well as maintaining friendships.

These are the most commonly encountered issues that we will discuss the best ways to tackle these issues in the next pages. There is a possibility of experiencing different issues, however they're usually a result of the base issues. For example, if your child is having trouble playing with toys or is extremely bossy and directive it is likely that he has difficulties sharing his thoughts with others. Once you've identified the social deficit or weaknesses your child is facing The subsequent step would be to deal with the issue using tried and tested strategies for education. This can include role-playing and play dates for practice, visual cues, as well as video examples.

If you are teaching your child about social skills It's crucial to keep in mind that you must not just teach them the techniques however, you must also explain the reason you're teaching them. Children are smarter than what parents believe. Unless you explain it to them and explain what it is that might offend them to not discuss an item with someone else and they may get angry and be quite difficult to deal with.

It is important to always be patient, and to be delicate and careful. Positive reinforcement can significantly simplify the process of teaching. In addition to its ability to boost confidence, it could also be a wonderful method of telling your child that they are improving.

The idea of enhancing interpersonal skills in the home

Making sure your child is taught social skills is a task that you must confine to your own home.

Family members such as godparents, grandparents as well as siblings can assist with their social development. It is important to play situations that are real and teach the children to behave as well as is possible. Just telling them what to do won't help as much as demonstrating them how to react visually.

Learning through examples and visual stimuli are always able to produce more effective outcomes. Therapists can also assist with play dates and role-playing. Experts and other outsiders are occasionally accepted, but it is suggested to reduce your physical involvement to the minimal level. Children who suffer from ASD tend to be afraid and intimidated or aggressive towards strangers. Make sure the circle is small.

Roleplaying

As we've already talked about the importance of visual stimulation. crucial, and nothing is so stimulating as reimagining possible scenarios, and encouraging your child to use the correct social abilities. Role-playing can be as simple as making up comfortable scenarios and helping them deal with it more effectively, or the introduction of a new or frightening situation and leading through the process.

You could, for instance, imagine that you're the same person as your child's closest friend at school. Or, pretend to be the dentist your child is afraid of visiting. In both scenarios you can have breaks and instruct your child what to do and to avoid doing. It's essential to provide a touch of adversary from time when you want to test him. When you play role-playing it is important to keep in mind that the situation gets more difficult before it improves. If you practice enough the child will soon be able to comprehend and learn how to manage challenging situations.

Video examples

Videos are a great way to teach social norms and signals like turning, non-verbal communication and sharing. You can stop the video to provide explanations at intervals of time about the exact nature of what's

21

happening between the people in the conversation . Then, you can clarify what should be considered appropriate and what is not.

It can also be a great method to teach children how to begin conversations, build acquaintances, and maintain friendships. Videos are frequently combined with role-playing. Videos can be used to help introduce concepts and reinforce them later through role-playing and acting exercises.

Visual cues

Visual cues are a popular and effective method of teaching the toddler to communicate nonverbally as well as effective social skills. It helps him recognize and prompt complex responses in the right situations. It also teaches him about conversational starting points. For instance, if they observe someone stretching their hands after making an introduction this could be an invitation to welcome them with a handshake. Additionally, a hand extended with an item such as a drink, food or food item that is of a certain kind could mean that they are inviting you to take a bite. A smile could be an indication of non-verbal communication that the person is seeking an apology or perhaps a gesture of compassion. A hand held out in the open could signal an invitation to hug, and holding a hand open in front of an individual's face could signal an indication of some sort.

Play dates for practice

Playdates with friends are the last phase of developing social abilities. They allow your child to apply every lesson, valuable knowledge, and skills you have helped him learn during your education. For instance, you could introduce your little one to the idea of boundary intrusion. You could also invite your best friend to learn a lesson from life with him. This adds a bit of variety into your regular lessons , and ensures that your child is developing as an individual.

Participating in games and other situations

The art of teaching non-verbal communication in conversation and keeping it up is something else, but actually beginning it is a different matter completely. It's crucial to teach your kids how to participate in discussions as effortlessly as is possible to ensure they get what they desire from every conversation. In order to instruct your child the basics of how to start and continue conversations they need to be taught by your child about the importance of conversational cues as well as the best conversation starters.

Conversation starters are concepts of images, thoughts, and comments that usually indicate a common characteristic or interest or characteristic. Conversation starters can be a bit tricky and can be difficult to understand them. However, with enough practice, they are learned and improved. The best topics or conversation starters are those that both speakers are familiar with. It could be everything from cooking to TV programs, or maybe Santa Claus. Conversation starters are considered offensive if they highlight the wrong or harmful behavior someone doesn't want to expose. For instance, someone who is addicted to alcohol might not want to hear you ask it out. Most of the time, the most appropriate conversational opener is typically the person's strengths or passion.

Conversational cues are verbal as well as non-verbal signals of a person's intent to keep or change the subject matter, or even end an ongoing conversation. As with the conversation starters they are sometimes difficult to learn or to master. Verbal expressions are among the most used signals. If a person announces through the use of speech that they must go, or asks to discuss something or another, they are expressing their wishes for the future. Learn your young children the meaning of conversations these words using one of the methods we've discussed previously.

Finding non-verbal cues is a more difficult task, particularly when they are related to conversational cues. They typically involve expressions or facial expressions. For example, if one's head is twitching or appears confused, it might be an ideal time to think about changing the subject. Moving backwards physically could indicate anxiety, or perhaps they're trying to signal that they're ready to leave. It is possible to teach your children about non-verbal communication cues making use of video examples or images.

Also, instruct them to observe pleasantries in conversations. It is important to teach them that it is important to share pleasantries while talking to strangers they are comfortable with. Discuss how they can effortlessly change conversations by recognizing the non-verbal and verbal signals in conversation and pick a topic they believe the other person will enjoy.

Loss and grief

Accepting loss of any kind is an essential aspect of growing older. Children may not be able to comprehend the concept of loss on a large scale but a gradual introduction of the notion is best for children, and especially those with ASD. If they learn to take losses in a smaller way at an earlier age, it is much easier to deal with it on a greater and more catastrophic scale.

Loss can take on any way. It doesn't need to be as serious such as losing the scientific fair an event; it may be a loss in something as simple as a match of tag. It's important to let people realize that everyone is going to have to lose.

The winners also lose And some of the greatest winners of history began as losers. The lesson is the perfect opportunity to introduce them to Abraham Lincoln. He was among the most successful presidents America ever had He was also the first president to start losing every single race he participated in. The president was an example of loss, you can teach your children about how to deal with loss. They will be teased and attempt to cause them to feel guilty about their own shortcomings. It is important to show children that it's important to feel confident no matter how bad kids appear.

It is possible to teach them mantras to repeat whenever they're likely to be annoyed. The mantras should include words or phrases that they trust or truly like. They should include things that help them stay focused on the positive side, feel secure as they remain grounded and encourage them to ignore bullies. Help them understand the importance of not doubting yourself because it's crucial in learning to handle loss. It is important to remind that small losses such as the loss at tag do not matter in the way that people think. The whole game is focused on having fun. Help them be focused on having fun, not winning. The less they focus on losing or winning the less upset they'll feel when they win or lose.

Social skills are hard to master, no matter what. It doesn't matter whether your child falls in the spectrum of autism or is not. Childhood is an extremely vulnerable time in the life of a child. It creates the foundation of a child's personality . It also determines aspects of their personality, preferences dislikes, likes and fears. The ability to teach children good social skills can help ease the pressure in this crucial stage of their growth.

Chapter 3: Communication

Communication is a fundamental human need that requires two or more individuals exchanging information using languages and other forms of communication. Communication doesn't require the use of words. Sometimes phrases, words, or even sentences can be classified as covert meanings that only those who have access to particular experiences are able to understand. Communication is vast and to fully comprehend it, it is necessary to examine concepts like semantics, semiotics and even pragmatics.

For children who have ASD Communication can be very complicated. It is not always the case that children with ASD are proficient in their speech or recognize non-verbal signals of communication in the same way as other children. As as a parent, it's crucial to get to grips with this. Be aware of your child's location on the spectrum and manage your expectations accordingly.

How do they communicate and grab your focus

The majority of people communicate both verbally and non-verbally. Most of the time verbal communication is by speaking using a widely used language, which is shared by the person speaking and by those listening. Additionally the verbal language isn't just limited to the languages. It can also involve spoken sounds. Babies, for instance, don't speak with any particular spoken language. They just make sounds and assume that their needs are acknowledged by their parents or caregivers.

Non-verbal communication is the process of communication that is not based on speech or sound. It's the process of transmitting information via eye contact or gestures, postures as well as visual cues and body language. The range of non-verbal communication is vast and absurd. There are an endless number of ways humans communicate. Many of them don't require sound or language whatsoever. Children who suffer from ASD mostly use spoken communication, and only a small amount of non-verbal communication to pass information. They have difficulty understanding subtle communication signals, which is usually the case when a communicator decides to switch to non-verbal communication. In some cases children who have ASD excel in regards to non-verbal communication, such as signs.

Every child has a distinct communication style. It's an integral element of their identity and it is important to recognize this distinctive pattern and be able to anticipate the meaning behind it. For instance, if your child is reciting certain words repeatedly and over again, it's that there is a reason behind it. This is known as echolalia and is extremely common in children with ASD. It can happen due to many reasons, and, in the majority of cases it's a means to tell you what they feel or what they are looking for. If your child continues to repeat the same phrase that he saw on TV and it's tied to something tangible, such as objects, the chances are that he's trying to convey to you that he would like this object.

Children who have ASD often use invented words and pronouns that switch. This is a normal method of getting around and eventually learning the language. As we've said earlier, it's crucial to know how to read between the line and be able to anticipate the needs of your child. Echolalia has been identified as the affluent communication disorder among children who suffer from ASD However, it's not all the way children express their emotions, needs or thoughts. It's no surprise that children also express their thoughts without speaking. They may express them as temper tantrums, anger or even repetitive behaviors. Like speaking, it's essential not to get caught up about how wrong your child's actions are or the impact it may affect your self-image. Instead, think about why your child took the action you did, and what the message he's trying to convey to you. If, for instance, your child is able to throw away a toy they do dislike, it might be due to it causing distress for the child or it is making him feel uncomfortable. Consider talking with him to find out the root of the issue. Understanding the inner workings of the mind of your child could be the key to a successful outcome down the road. Assistive devices can also be considered an avenue for communication. Children with limited language control may be able to take a shortcut using an assistive device to explain exactly what he requires. There are beautiful images within these apps to signify needs or actions. When your child clicks them, parents or guardians can instantly determine what the child is in need of.

Support communication development

It's well-known that children who have autism experience issues with the development of their communication abilities. They require constant support and assistance to ensure that they don't fall behind in particular areas. Communication is considered to be an essential part of survival in many societies. Having a lack of control over your abilities to communicate can be viewed as a significant disadvantage. As parents, it is your obligation to ensure that your child's communication skills to the best of his abilities. Let's take a look at the methods you can use to encourage great growth in communication.

One of them is communicating through examples. Children learn best by imitating. They will imitate you once they observe how you speak or behave in a certain manner. When you speak be sure to use the correct words and use appropriate gestures. After having seen it several times, they'll be able to connect gestures, words or movements to specific objects or concepts. Children who use non-verbal communication their primary means of communication should teach sign language, paying particular attention paid to gestures as well. It's crucial not to miss any step of the communicative process. Because the majority of sign language uses hand gestures, you need to always correct your mistakes and make the correct gestures constantly.

Incorporate communicative media into the curriculum and help them learn new skills every now and then. Although a child's brain is basically one of informational sponges, it requires some guidance. As you limit your child's vocabulary of specific words and add others later You should also teach communication skills similarly. Learn tablets and apps in this effort. There are many great learning apps that can simplify the process of learning and make it easier for your children. You want them to fully master an existing skill before introduction to a new or more complicated technique.

Allow your child to get some actual-world training every once in awhile. The sole reason to teach your child advanced communications or language skills is to make sure that they is able to use them in the proper context within the actual world. The world of the real is more calming when you teach your child that it's. Begin by gently weaning him, and let him speak whenever you go to the doctor or the restaurant.

Also, alter the context when you can. The world is vast and diverse. In the majority of cases the examples in the textbooks you've worked through with your child thousands of times will not be what is presented to him when he's communicating. As a coach for communicative communication, you should be aware that communication is highly contextual and that different situations require different strategies. It's difficult to think of all possible scenarios in which the phrase could be used in however, you can take steps to minimize confusion for your child. It is possible to shake things up often and introduce new areas as well as people, times, and locations as you play.

A significant part of growing your child up is the process of learning and expanding as your child grows and develops. As as a parent, you need to not be confused when your child is doing some thing or gets behind in a particular way. You should be at the top of your game in order to keep on top of your child's development and development.

How do you motivate them to speak up

Inspiring them to utilize languages and other methods of communication isn't just an effective way to enhance their skills in speaking however, it's also an excellent way to help people overcome their anxiety. The only way in which language abilities can be improved is to utilize the language as often as you can. Children who suffer from ASD tend to be quiet about their own. They are scared that people will not understand them, and so they prefer not to talk even once. As their guardian and friend try to encourage them to be more open to the world by introducing them to issues that they have expressed an interest in. It is possible to use positive reinforcement to encourage them to build confidence in their communication or language abilities. It is essential to attempt to encourage them to communicate as often as you can. Talk to them about their day, what they enjoy or who they've had conversations with. All of these will give them the training they require to meet their goals in interaction in the future.

Imitating their behavior and speech patterns is a kind of positive reinforcement that has its roots in psychology of behavior. If you demonstrate to the children how stylish their features or sounds are, they're less likely to question themselves in the future. It also encourages continuous involvement, and could be a marker of correction to indicate the moment they've strayed from the acceptable norm. As an example, suppose it's a game in which you and your child continuously imitate each other. When you stop, they'll observe and guess that the reason is due to unacceptable behaviour. Inviting your child to speak through direct questions and providing them with non-verbal cues is a particularly effective method to get them to talk or talk more. When you ask them these questions, you're giving them the opportunity to speak and put the information they've acquired to use.

Maintaining a language that is simple and entertaining is a fast and efficient method to keep them engaged. Communicating concepts and speaking in terms they can comprehend can encourage them to keep talking since they feel they're speaking to someone who understands. The complexities of language and the big words can be intimidating regardless of what age your child may be and you should always have them with you while you talk. It is also possible to keep them talking and excited when you talk about the subject they are fascinated by. Every kid has a toy, cartoon or cartoon that they cannot stop talking about. Once you've identified the thing that your child is most interested in discuss it in detail.

Furthermore, it is recommended that you allow therapists to do some of the heavy lifting for you. It is tempting to attempt to handle everything yourself. Therapists are professionals specially trained to help you and your children with their communication issues. It is helpful to let them perform their work and then take some time to yourself. Children, generally, often create walls around themselves. They may be wary of strangers, and may are able to isolate themselves from others if they don't feel at ease. As a caregiver it's essential to ensure that you do not let your child grow into shy or introverted in this early age. The communication skills of their children may suffer and they'll face difficult time integrating into the society. It's crucial to break through that wall through role-playing as well as imitation, love and a jolly conversation every time you are able to.

Chapter 4: The Building Of Fun Routines

Being a parent to an autistic child could be extremely challenging and, at times it can be stressful. It is important to get the most out of it and view the experience as something more rather than an obligation. Children are gifts and having fun and engaging practices can help make the process of raising them infinitely enjoyable for all those who is involved.

Routines are a series of coordinated activities that are often repeated at predetermined intervals. They should be specific, organized and a little flexible. They are tightly planned and usually repeated after a certain period of time. They are utilized to handle complicated and delicate events or objects. Children are among the most complex and delicate creatures on the planet and require a strong routine to succeed. A single mistake could permanently ruin your day and waste time that you don't need.

Create a fun routine that you Will Be able to Maintain

They are designed to last and be long-term in usage. This means you need to create the kind of routine you are able to follow with no ambiguity. There are several points to consider when you plan to sketch out an initial routine.

It is important to be very cautious in your time-allocations and daily objectives. In attempting to do more than one thing can lead to spillovers that result in your routine falling off the rails. The idea of trying to do it right the first time to build the routine is rather naive. Like many people, the best method can only be discovered through trial and trial and. Don't get discouraged when the plan doesn't work in a flash. Instead, make some time and learn every success.

Your schedule should begin early in the morning, and then end at the time your child goes to bed. Children are usually active during the daytime. Therefore, you must ensure that you include this in your daily routine. Plan a more time aside to do your daily tasks in the morning to give yourself the cushion to deal with those unexpected, unplanned outbursts.

For tasks like preparing for school or eating breakfast require additional time. Ten minutes should suffice. However, don't be afraid to extend the time If your child needs it.

Additionally, you should allow for a few lessons when you're making your schedule. The ability of children to master certain skills improves through practice It is advisable to plan time for basic as well as more complicated communicative classes all throughout your working day. It's impossible to predict when you'll have to present long lessons on specific concepts. They usually require you to instruct them right away while the event is present in your kid's brain. If you are taking too long to prepare you could miss out on the chance. While you may not be able to anticipate these kinds of situations however, you can certainly prepare in case they pop up. And they will.

Make use of a vision board to try out your possible routines

One way to cut the learning curve by half and putting together your first routine that is functional is to create different scenarios in your head. It is essential to make frequent hypotheses and play a variety of scenarios inside your head. You know what you must accomplish during the day. You know the personality of your child and the way he reacts to certain events. You can make a schedule and then imagine how it will play out. If you plan it correctly you will be able to immediately see what could fail. After that, you can add a time-span to see how it could improve the situation. You could also shift things around by putting one thing after another.

Making adjustments to routines that are unexpected

It's possible to sketch or plan out a close to perfect system that will work for the majority of the times. However, it is impossible to find a solution that works every day. Change is inevitable and people who are adults tend to embrace change with wide arms. However, it can be a bit scary for children with autism. The unknowing is often connected to risk and it is important to do to be as normal as possible by preparing yourself and your child for the event or the change that's to occur. Imagine yourself in the shoes of your child and think about how he would react to the situation and then utilize the responses you gather to plan the actual occasion.

There are two common methods of handling a possibly triggering event. One of them is the one we've just mentioned that allows you to be taught to anticipate frightening and exciting events and also take care of damage control. This approach involves teaching your child to anticipate trigger events and demonstrate the normality of these things. The best way to help normalize the triggering events is by introducing them to them in a positive and non-threatening manner. It is possible to do this using a storyboard, or a visual aid. It is possible to swap objects using a photo of the items and then create a slide outlining the advantages and benefits of these ideas or ideas.

The second approach is dealing with the consequences of these encounters by explaining the situation in the moment and instructing your child to not be scared of it. Make sure you create a specific routine to help them cope with an unexpected change that they do not fully comprehend. Making a calm routine they can go through when they're feeling overwhelmed may aid in preventing outbursts and screaming before they happen. For instance an unexpected visit to the emergency room could be extremely frightening and complicated. It's normal that your child will respond by crying and throwing an angry tantrum. It is possible to calm him with a request to start an calming routine that you have tried repeatedly over again. Rehearsing various techniques for controlling emotions prior to any frightening or difficult changes is a great method to assist your child adjust to the new world that he's just was exposed.

As parents, you are aware that children won't behave in a way without a valid justification, even if that just doesn't seem to make sense to you. In public, tantrums and explosions indicate something more serious and uncomfortable. To effectively deal with sudden anger, it is important to take advantage of your child's connection to the things they love most. They can serve as comfort toys for your child. Items like headphones, sunglasses and other toys could be a great way to ease the pain they are experiencing and could help defuse the situation before it becomes out of control. Exercises that calm them are also great ways to assist them in handling stressful situations. Activities such as nature walks and yoga can be a good way to teach them how to be calm and under control. In addition breathing exercises are an effective strategy to control their anger or reactions.

Sometimes , when children behave or show fear what they really need is to feel safe and loved. You'll be amazed at how effective the presence of a parent and their love can be during sensitive times. The importance of empathy is when trying to stop noisy and public anger. Inflicting punishment on them can only make the situation worse. You must show compassion and offer them the exact things you'd like should you be in their position.

While both are excellent as a pair, as a pair, they're not the ideal way to handle potentially frightening and stressful situations. The best option is using a combination of both strategies. If the lessons don't connect with your child You can always help be able to calm them afterward.

The planning for changes that are expected to occur in routines

Change comes in many kinds of shapes and dimensions and doesn't have to be a major event or life-changing. It could be like a simple change in a cereal brand. But it could also be that is as significant as going to the new school. 9 out of 10 times children who suffers from ASD is likely to find any new change and even small changes to routines extremely frightening which is the reason it is important to be prepared and manage the reactions of your child.

It's possible to calm his fears by re-normalizing the whole experience by telling stories. A narrative about your experience during that particular experience can help bring your child to a calmer place. If, for instance, you're planning to visit a physician with your kid, you can tell him a story of the experience you had with the doctor and how they helped you, even if it was somewhat frightening initially.

Create a visual schedule that alerts them to any sudden changes. Even if it's unexpected and unintentional, watching it come closer to each other every day could get your child used to the changes and make it easier for them to accept. It is recommended to invest in a stunning graphic calendar that allows them to actually see the events of the coming weeks before they happen and make themselves ready for this experience. You can also make an individual calendar. If you're not able to find one that has the theme your child enjoys, making your own calendar gives you the freedom to do whatever you'd like to do with it. It might seem like an arduous and difficult process however, it could be worth it. It's as easy as speaking with a graphic designer about what you need to accomplish.

The introduction of a new thing can be less challenging and stressful for your child if you give him plenty of time to process and adjust to the new or alteration. It is possible to show him images of what is expected to occur at the new school, institute or appointment. It is crucial to allow your child to moderately normalize the events set to take place. The longer time your child is given to react more fully, the more time they have to react. Changes don't have to be scary and can be very exciting as well. Your child could be in love with a brand new sport or activity you've just been introduced to. This is more frequent than you imagine and can be controlled effectively through the introduction of a timer, and instructing your child to follow the timer. When you hear the timer going off it could be an indication that you need to stop what you're doing.

Modifying your schedule slowly instead of abruptly will teach your child to be able to handle change in a controlled way. Perhaps you're planning to help your child to become a bit more independent by teaching the proper way to brush his teeth. You can gradually get his teeth ready by letting him brush his teeth.

The change in your schedule isn't always terrifying or thrilling but it can also be boring. But, you can help your children to be more accepting of the new, seemingly boring schedule by tying it to something that they are interested in. You can also create excitement through incentives and praise to inspire to get them involved. Making changes to your routine requires much effort, time and meticulous planning. You must take extra care when planning an individual change in routine and attempt to anticipate your little child's reaction and prepare for it with care. The change in your schedule doesn't need to be a complicated process. It's simple and straightforward. It can also be delightfully effortless.

Reward flexibility

Routine creates structure and helps children with autism to maintain control over various aspects that affect their daily lives. It can be extremely beneficial and help them stay grounded and calm for the majority all the time. It can, however it could be a hindrance. It is crucial to help them understand the value of flexibility and the benefits that go with it. As parents should your child be taught how to adapt, it means you will have less public drama and reduce your time. This could be beneficial for your child. It allows them to face challenging and new situations with less anxiety and greater control. This will greatly enhance their social skills as well as reduce the fear that they have of being in the unknowing.

The advantages of flexibility are enormous. As parents, it provides you more confidence and comfort that your child will be a good person in public settings. However, it can also aid in establishing control and order in your things your child is involved in. If you have a child, the ability to be flexible is an essential step to take. Once he has achieved it you, you can move to more advanced and higher ones. This basically boosts his growth.

It is important to realize that encouraging your child to accept flexible doesn't mean you allow him to experience unfamiliar and frightening situations. It is possible to begin with a positive attitude and reward your child every time he does something unique or is doing something new. You can give him more time for play or increasing the amount of time he spends on gadgets or by giving him nutritious snacks.

Things to avoid in the event that your kid is throwing a fit because he's scared

A situation is likely to occur sooner or later for children who have autism. As an adult, you've probably had a similar experience. It's different based the mood of your child, however, it is likely to involve various shouts, cries and sometimes even throwing toys. If it's caused by the fear of or discomfort There are a variety of ways you can try to stop it.

The first thing you must be wary of is making a loud noise at him. When your child throws an angry fit in public, because of fear and is frightened, the first thing you should shout at him. The only thing you'll be doing is inflaming the situation and making it more difficult to deal with in the future. The other thing you should avoid is getting nervous. If you are anxious during a meltdown, it can cloud your thoughts and make it difficult to decide on the worst solution to the issue your child is suffering.

Thirdly, don't get embarrassed. Yes, it is quite embarrassing to confront your child's rage in public. However, it is important to keep in mind the fact that you are the one who is in discomfort, not the other bystanders. They're just spectators and they aren't important to you as far as they are concerned. Concentrate on your child and let everyone rant and complain all they'd like.

Last but not least, remember to reward him once you see him calm down in the end. Children react more positively to rewards than they do to punishment. Make sure to show them you appreciate their efforts by rewarding their effort accordingly. Making a schedule that your child can follow is a crucial aspect of being a parent. It might take some time or testing however, you'll find it in the end. Once you've done that it, the job will be much more straightforward.

Chapter 5: Parent's Manual

So far the book has been mostly focused on children with autism. We've discussed helping them overcome their greatest concerns and weaknesses, but we haven't focused on parents, guardians or anyone else who is faced with having a child with autism. According to the CDC states that 1 out of eighty families has one or more children with autism. This means that across America families across the country must deal with this new reality with no prior notification or preparation.

The new information could be extremely challenging and frightening. It's enough to break families and force children to grow up in broken families. It's not uncommon for parents break up because of the strain of parenting children generally. When you add the burden of the responsibility of caring for a child diagnosed with autism it's an issue that many would prefer to stay clear of. As parents, you're required handle whatever challenges come to you with no any hesitation or slowing down however, humans aren't only built to be like that. It is important to take the time to think about everything you are learning to prepare your self for the long path ahead, not believing that everything is going to be fine. This chapter we'll be looking at parents and guardians who are facing changes. We'll discuss ways you can manage the diagnosis and raising children with autism.

Reaction to the diagnostic

Parents with no idea about autism will likely to be the most affected by the information. Parents are usually scared and upset when they discover the fact that their children were born with a disorder that has been viewed as a stigma for a long time. However, it's not as restrictive or difficult as you think it is. Although it is difficult to accept and acknowledge it is important to acknowledge this and be careful not to experience a complete crying in the doctor's office when you realize the fact that you're set to alter forever. Certain things will change, but some aspects will stay the same.

You are still yours and any disorder shouldn't make you see your child in a different way.

Autism can cause communication difficulties for children, however it isn't necessary to be that way. New research centers, colleges and institutes devoted to helping children with autism have sprung in recent times across the world. There has been more progress over the last twenty years than was made over the past century. There's never been a more ideal time for your child's arrival to the world, as it is now, because there are ample resources to help you raise your child with the best manner feasible. Relax because it's not will be nearly as difficult as you imagine. With the right support and the right environment your child can lead an active, healthy, and fulfilling life.

When you realize that all the assistance you'll ever require is right there waiting for you The following step will be to figure out what sort of help you'll need for your particular situation. There are millions of excellent medical professionals as well as schools and specialists waiting to help you. The only way to fully take advantage of these new opportunities is to ensure you're fully informed. Make sure you do a lot of study and study the various terms as well as laws and rights. It is important to research terms such as personalized learning programs for children, least restrictive environments earlier intervention Individuals with Disabilities Education Act, Free and Appropriate Public Education and others. Find out what's best and what is not. Study journals and get immersed in the available literature. Find websites on the internet or join support forums that you believe will aid you.

Therapists and neurologists agree that the early years are most critical for a child with autism. The brain is malleableand lots of progress is possible during that time. In these crucial years, it's crucial to get him every assistance you can get. Make a team of doctors and make appointments with specialists and therapy professionals who are at high levels in their field. Additionally, you'll require the assistance of other specialists in your field like neurologists, pediatricians and psychical therapists, biomedical experts as well as speech and language therapists. Always consult with all of these experts when you think you may require them, and ensure that you keep the relationship lively and healthy.

The raising of an autistic child can be an enjoyable and transformational experience. It makes you step beyond your comfort zone and grow as an individual. Being a parent of an autistic child often involves becoming a professional therapist yourself. Simple and effective methods of therapy such as the Applied Behavior Analysis, The Floortime Method and the fast methods of prompting as well as The Picture Exchange Communication System, the Verbal Behavior Analysis, and the method of a sensory diet are just a few innovative and fascinating techniques you could need to acquire to assist your child deal with his communication and social challenges. The methods of therapy listed here are only a few of the most well-known methods of teaching. Employing only one method is not recommended. There are many strategies available and it is important to take advantage of the many sources and information that are available. They may be the best way to overcome the latest hurdles in your child's communication.

Finding the top doctors as well as specialists and therapists isn't going to cost a lot. A very crucial aspects of the process of preparing and reacting is to create an appropriate financial plan for you. The estimates suggest that the care of an individual with autism throughout their entire life could cost around $3 million dollars. That is much more than what families can earn over the course of 10 years. This cost can be very heavy for a household, specifically when only one parent is employed. It is suggested that families that aren't financially able to pay for the costs without a budget should look to the government or great insurance plans to ease the burden. There are a variety of assistance laws as well as benefits available to families living in more than 25 states across America. Parents and caregivers should consider reducing costs by reducing expenses that they could learn to eliminate. The key point to consider to remember is that budgeting for finances is a crucial and challenging aspect of planning your future life as parents. It is a very stressful and demoralizing experience, and it's best to start immediately.

If you are a parent of a child who has autism, it is important to keep a record of your child's development. Being a parent of a child who has autism can be challenging and exhausting. Sometimes, the difficulties can lead you to focus the negative aspect of your child's life. That's why keeping a log of your child's progress and treatment plans is crucial. Not only can it serve as an indicator of the way you and your child have progressed as well as providing the information you'll require in the future. From where you're at it's difficult going through the motions and transforming from panic to keeping a diary. When you transition from being shocked to being proactive parents it is crucial to remember where you came from. A proper first reaction is vital and you should be aware that your choice and attitude should not stop your child from receiving the assistance he requires.

Your parental role

Some people might believe that you're lucky or that you are a bit naive at first of discovering your child's diagnosis However, you do have an obligation as parent. Yes, it's much more challenging to parent a child who has autism. However, you're still a parent, and you are obligated to fulfill certain duties which you need to fulfill.

The first one is the job as a caretaker. As parents, you're an automatic caretaker. You're the one who is responsible for the joyous bundle you refer to as your child. The responsibility of the caregiver is magnified when you have an autistic child. The expense of care rises and you must be prepared for the never-ending medical expenses that he'll have to pay throughout his life. It is essential to prepare for the increased cost. It is your responsibility to take care of any medical and nutritional requirements that your client may have.

It's not obvious however, you're actually your child's best friend. Nobody else will be more present for him as you do. As his closest friend you have to learn how to be sensitive to his needs for emotional support and be focused on understanding and supporting him. As his most trusted friend it is your responsibility to introduce him terrifying and new concepts. It can become an overwhelming and scary making introductions a challenge, but preparing for them can make it more manageable for the child.

You also are the resident authority persona. Parents often assume that their autistic children's needs and wants are a given. They can be spoiled and don't hesitate to tell them"no" every once in time. Children with autism are still children. They might not be able to communicate in the way you're familiar with but they are communicating the same. As parents, it is not a good idea to overindulge your child by offering him everything he desires. The effect will be similar to giving the child everything he wants for regardless of whether he really require it. The child will be unjust and disrespectful. As a parent, your responsibility is to raise your child in a respectful manner and firmly, saying no is the best way to do this. Make sure to tell them no time. This will help them become less dependent, and also teach them a bit about how things work in the real world.

Dealing with the circumstances

Do you realize that most parents have difficulty to accept their children have autism? It's much easy to accept that it's just a phase that your child will eventually overcome. However it's a permanent condition and your child will need to be a part of it throughout his life. As parents, must deal with it. It can take a long time for most people to truly accept their new reality. certain people are not being able to comprehend or accept it.

The majority of parents blame it on their genes , or blame it on their parenting. They think it's all their fault that they didn't give enough time during the initial few months of their child's development, or due to an autism history within their families or something similar to that. They believe it's necessary to blame someone else or something that is tangible. They also often feel an overwhelming sense of loss and may even grieve their child as if they passed away and then reincarnated as another person.

Some parents completely deny the child they are raising is autistic. They decide to seek an opinion from a different source and consult as many specialists and doctors as they can. They are looking for someone to lie to them and assure them that everything will be fine. No matter what class you could fall into when you learn about your child's behavior is important to be grieving.

The word "grief" doesn't necessarily mean that you're mourning your child. It's actually more about accepting the fact that your child isn't the person you believed you were. It's about actively making an effort to accept the new reality you're facing as a parent for the first time. The process involves letting go of what you believed was you and becoming who your kid wants to be. The grieving process is typically the experience of fear and denial, sadness, and even anger. All of these feelings are normal as part of the grieving process. The most important thing is that you feel all of those frightening emotions and let them go by grieving.

When you are grieving While you grieve, remember that autism is not a problem. There's no problem for your child. It's not a curse or unlucky luck or anything like that. It shouldn't lead you to be apathetic to your children as you're always focussed on one. Your other children should receive the same amount of love like your child with autism. We'll discuss more details about balancing your caregiving duties between those children later in chapter 9.

It is different for every person. Some people simply rub it on and then slap it off, while other find themselves grieving much longer. The majority of people fall into the second group. It's fine to take time to fully comprehend the new reality. The most important thing is that you're trying to accept the new reality.

How can you avoid stress and take good care of yourself

Have a day off for yourself every now and again. Parents are often told that they do not have time off, but they ought to. Being concerned and caring about your kids can become exhausting after a couple of months of no enough rest. It is a good idea to take a rest day occasionally to relax and find your rhythm. If you have a child who has autism, it does not mean that he is your whole world. A little separation can benefit each of us.

If you are in a committed partnership; you can let your spouse steer the wheel for a few hours or so. It doesn't need to be an extended vacation, it must be enough to let you relax. A trip with your family can be a great method of taking care of your family and yourself while having fun. A getaway to a cabin, or summer house can be an excellent opportunity to take your child out of the pollution and noise of the city. In this time you can concentrate on their communication skills and social skills. Relaxing by frequent trips for a spa day is an excellent way to relax. A day spent with your loved ones doing something you like is an additional beneficial activity that you ought to do frequently. It may not be as relaxing like taking an unplanned sabbatical, however it can work just as well.

You can also consider an activity. Hobbies are low-cost stress-reducing activities which can assist in cooling down after a hard and tiring day. The pursuit you select can be whatever. It is also possible to have an occasional passion time. Parents have their preferred accessory or comfort item. For some, it's food, other parents, drinks. Whatever you prefer to wear as your personal comfort device be sure to count on it whenever you're feeling overwhelmed or feel like treating yourself to a treat. A little self-care can go a very long way.

Chapter 6: Helping Your Child Who Has Autism

To Thrive

Making sure your child is successful is a crucial aspect of caring for a child with autism. Parents must make specific adjustments for their children who are autistic as their growth patterns aren't going to follow the usual way of life. This will require coming up with new ways to connect with the child. This can be very difficult if you've had other children who did not have ASD. However, all it takes is the knowledge of a new method of conducting things. It's possible to imagine it as parenting 2.0. Apart from learning to speak, you'll have to create a space that allows your child to be at ease to express himself and play without danger of injuries. This includes childproofing your home and taking few additional safety security measures.

Following your consultation to the doctor, and any subsequent diagnosis, you'll likely receive some type of guidance about what to do next.

This includes aiding you in finding support and assistance and establishing your treatment strategy. This chapter covers each of these issues in great detail. Let's start with one of the most crucial factors, i.e. creating structure and security.

Create structure and ensure safety

We'll begin by addressing the issue of structure. Even if you're the same new to managing the autism spectrum as your kid but you shouldn't take this as an excuse. If you're planning to offer the structure that your child needs, you'll need to be as knowledgeable possible about autism. This has been discussed in earlier chapters. Once you've mastered the issue, you can develop the habit of being consistent.

Consistency is among the most crucial strategies you can offer your child. The reason for this is that children who suffer from ASD typically have difficulty in transferring lessons from one area to the next. Therefore, if your child is learning something at school, implementing the same lesson at home will not be easy. One of the most common examples is signing language. Children who have ASD might learn the basics at school, but they never consider using it at home to communicate. This is concerned with keeping the child engaged in the process of learning. It is essential to know what your child is learning at the classroom or in the therapist's office and figure out an opportunity to apply the methods at home.

Another tip is to allow your child to be a part of a variety of environment. If you're having sessions with a doctor's office, you can schedule one at your home. The change in the environment can help your child transfer knowledge and skills from one situation or setting to another.

Another essential aspect of providing structure to your child is creating and adhering to a routine. Children who suffer from ASD thrive in highly controlled environments. The predictable and routine nature of their everyday tasks will help them remain focus. Your schedule should contain time for meals and therapy sessions and school hours, playtime and even bedtime.

The key is to regularity. You must adhere to your schedule if it's likely to work. Try to limit disruptions to a minimal. Do away with them completely as much as you are able to. If you notice that disruption will occur, try to prepare your child for disruption ahead of time and attempt to adapt it to the system. We've already talked about this in detail within chapter 4. It is a good reference to learn more or as an overview.

The next aspect of the topic of setting up a structure is rewarding the good behaviour. Positive reinforcement is crucial in the care of children who have ASD. Therefore, one of your obligations will be to be observant of good actions that your child performs. Even if it was not intended, praises can inspire the child to do it again. Other rewards could include letting your child play with their favorite toy or handing the child stickers.

Now, let's talk about the issue of safety. In the past, we talked about the ways that raising a child with autism is similar to being a parent 2.0. Similar to this, as providing a secure living space will outshine any child-proofing that you've done before. However, this does not mean that you don't require the most basic measures to protect your children, such as placing dangerous substances and products on shelves high, or protecting electrical outlets.

Other safety measures include protecting your windows in the form of replacing your glass Plexiglas which is a stronger alternative that is shatter-proof and durable. It is also recommended to install alarms and locks on every door you can. This is particularly crucial if your child is inclined to wander around. Installing alarms and locks will stop your child from wandering off and will notify you when they do this. As aspect of the parental 2.0 security measures, you must notify the local police and fire department about the tendency of your child to run away. Inform them about the ASD as well as any other accommodation the child and you require.

Find non-verbal ways to connect

The most challenging part of caring for a child with ASD is communicating with your child. However, the best part is you do not need to speak in order to communicate to your child. simple non-verbal signals, such as your gaze towards your kid, how you hold your child's hand, and even the sound of your voice can be able to communicate for you. As parents you are constantly speaking to you through a distinct way, even if you might not be aware of it. Enhancing the quality of your communication can be as easy as understanding the language your child uses and then letting them know that you are on the same page.

Your child may be able to communicate in subtle manners through body language and facial expressions. Pay attention to the sounds your child produces when he is hungry or is hungry or is exhausted. It is also important to discover the reasons behind the things you observe him doing. Like any child they are likely to have a temper tantrum and you'll need to deal with it. Children who have ASD can be misguided due the way they talk and therefore they are likely to be annoyed or angry more frequently.

This lack of understanding most of the time can result in the child throwing a tantrum. Similar to behavior of most children in general, children with ASD can throw a tantrum to draw attention and get an idea across. Learning to recognize the non-verbal signals they are sending is an excellent way to keep these tantrums at bay. If you recall from Chapter 1, we talked about the reason children do the things they do. Sometimes it's an appeal for assistance. Sometimes it's just your child trying to get your attention and you're not receiving the message. The temper tantrum could be an expression of anger. Being aware of this can help increase communication between you.

As we discussed the timetable we talked about creating an opportunity for having entertainment. Children in a home with ASD are still kids, and therefore, they're bound to want to play with their hearts to the max. It's important to create a space that allows your child to do it as easily and comfortably as they can. It isn't possible to fill your days with lessons and therapy sessions. It will only hinder the natural expression of your child. When you are creating a schedule the play time is best positioned around the time where your child is alert and awake. You want your child to have the most fun within the time frame.

When you are playing together with your kid, you can figure out new ways to keep him smiling and laughing. Do not try to incorporate classes or therapy in your play time, since your child will enjoy more when it's not another lesson. Playtime can be extremely beneficial to your kid. It can aid in connecting with your child in new and often surprising ways.

A very prevalent signs that children have ASD is heightened sensibility to sensory stimuli. You must pay close attention to determine whether your child suffers from any of these sensitivities. Sound, light, smell as well as taste all can cause discomfort. In other situations children suffering from ASD have less sensitivity to these triggers and require more stimulation if they will be able to identify these triggers.

Find out how stimuli affect the behavior of your child. Be aware of the ones which trigger positive reactions and those that provoke an unfavourable reaction. What are the triggers that cause stress and which are relaxing? If you know these issues, you'll be able to communicate with and bond to your kid in a better manner. It'll be much easier to pinpoint the cause of any problems that your child may have.

Develop a customized autism treatment strategy

Another crucial aspect to help your child succeed is to seek the right treatment. This is a crucial step as treatment sessions are intended to be an ongoing aspect of your child's existence. There are so many options for treatment that deciding on the best one can be a daunting task. The more difficult part is that everyone will attempt to offer some type of advice on the best method to approach your treatment. There's a good chance that you'll receive contradictory advice from your friends or teachers, as well as doctors. It is crucial to be aware that there's not a specific treatment program that's appropriate for all children with ASD. The most effective treatment is usually an amalgamation of several different activities. It must be determined by the uniqueness of your child. The method of treatment must take into account your child's interests, strengths and weaknesses.

There are a variety of factors an appropriate autism treatment plan should be able to consider. The treatment should be based upon your child's strengths, and must provide an outline that is dependable and achievable. It should also begin by giving your child a set of basic tasks that are divided into stages. Whatever strategy you decide on, you should also involve your child in regular positive reinforcements. Also, no treatment plan is sufficient in the absence of a plan to fully involve you with the child's treatment.

It's best to get to know your child's needs to a certain extent before you decide on the treatment strategy. This is because you'll need to answer the most basic questions about your child's behavior and then use the results to create a treatment plan that is tailored to your child's needs. Questions such as "What do you know about your child's talents?" "What behaviors are most annoying for you and your child?" "What skills does your child have the least?" "What's the most efficient method for your child to develop?" and of course, "What does your child like doing?" Any treatment plan that takes these factors into consideration is likely to be effective.

Apart from asking questions related to your child and you You should also ask questions related to treatment. Contact any treatment specialists you can find feasible and conduct a thorough quantity of study. The treatment plan must be oriented towards achieving goals, which is what helps you make the right decisions for you. It is not necessary to pick the most effective treatment option. So long as it is addressing the needs of your child You can mix several therapies.

A few of the most commonly used treatments include the play-based approach to therapy occupational therapy the therapy of speech and language and nutrition therapy. It is evident that no one therapy in this list can meet all your child's requirements. Thus, it is necessary to utilize a variety of different therapies for the most effective outcomes. In conclusion, in this area, you should not create a treatment plan that isn't viable. Your child's schedule shouldn't be filled with things they aren't interested in or cannot accomplish regularly. In order to not overwhelm your child, think about break up the sessions. Concentrate on learning the basics which are crucial first, then you'll be able to manage the rest later.

Get help and assistance

Parenting is, without doubt one of the most challenging jobs that you can have in the entire world. Being a parent of one who suffers from ASD is often twice as stressful as normal parenting. The process of watching your child's behavior, interpreting clues, and sticking to a set schedule may take lots of energy and time. It's common for parents to feel overwhelmed on number of days. Therefore, it's essential to take the time to look after yourself. You'll only be able to provide your child the best treatment when you're physically and mentally in good state. It's not a good idea to try to accomplish everything by yourself. It's not necessary to. It's obvious that taking responsibility for a kid suffering from ASD is a huge undertaking and seeking assistance is the only way to go. In fact, it's advised.

There are a variety of possibilities you have to take advantage of as parents in the event of needing assistance and support. You can go to ADS group support, as an instance. ADS support groups offer an excellent opportunity to meet and socialize with families similar to you are. It is possible to share information, tips and experiences with one another. Other families will be there for you to provide assistance and support when you require it. Additionally, you will have the chance to provide assistance parents who recently have had a diagnosis. Being aware of what they're struggling with could provide courage for them.

Another source of help you should consider can be respite services. There are many facilities that provide the opportunity to provide respite care to parents with autistic children. In the respite program, you'll allow another caregiver to look after your child for a short period of the time, providing you with time to rest and recuperate.

As parent, you're eligible for therapy and counseling. If you're worried that the task of taking care of your child is taking too much of your time might want to consult a therapist of your own. Therapy allows you to be honest and talk about the way you feel as well as your anxieties, fears and even your fears. It is also possible to seek counseling for family issues that you are experiencing within your own relationships. In the end, taking care of the child who is autistic is just equally your responsibility, just as the obligation of all members of your family.

If you are somewhere in the United States, your child will also be able to receive assistance by utilizing the Early Intervention Program. This program is offered to children as young as the age of 2. Before you are eligible for treatment through the Early Intervention Program, your child will need to undergo a no-cost evaluation. If the assessment uncovers a developmental issue The program's specialists can assist you in developing an individualized treatment plan. For children older than three years old help is provided through programs that are based at schools. They may be put in groups with children who are not developing properly.

Chapter 7: Practical Solutions To Everyday

Issues

In the past, we've discussed a lot of the topics that you must know as a parent of autism-related children. This chapter we'll try explore the practical issues you'll likely face each day, and possibly solutions. These are the kinds of issues that traditional parenting advice won't aid you in. For instance, eating and sleeping. Children with ASD may be very selective regarding their food. They may be more picky than children who are not autistic. You must be able to use all the knowledge you've learned for handling the issue. You shouldn't have to be able to tell them that you don't have to yell at them or say that they must eat it simply because you've told them that way.

Similar to issues with sleep. A schedule doesn't suffice for your child to fall asleep. There's a good chance that your child isn't understanding the idea behind an agenda. It's your job to ensure that the plan is strictly adhered to. Let's look at some of the issues you might encounter along with practical solutions to address them.

Food

A few children who have ASD have a very limited range of their diet choices. They may only choose between two or three options. Unfortunately all of them could be feasible in terms of diet. You'll recall that nutritional therapy is an integral component of the treatment plan for children suffering from ASD. The limited list of dietary options presents you with a problem.

The first step is to cut off the issue in the early stages. If you see that your child is progressively refusing any food item, you must to stop this trend as soon as you can. If you don't, your child may reduce the variety of food choices to a small number of unhealthy choices. If you allow this to happen, it's going to be harder to encourage your child to eat nutritious food choices. To begin the process, you must begin by selecting foods that are closest to your child's tastes. For example, if you find that your child is not able to eat an entire meal with strawberry ice cream it is best to start with feeding them strawberries. In some other cases it is possible that it is the appearance of food that could matter more than taste. For instance, if your child is fond of potato chips, then add corn chips into the food to replicate the texture.

You're likely to be concerned about the nutritional needs that your kid is getting. If that's the scenario, it is recommended to provide your child with multivitamins. They could provide additional nutrients that your child is lacking in the diet of corn chips.

In the next step, you'll have to start taking baby steps to introduce the child food items. This is vital since children with autism can be highly resistant to food changes. The best first step is to simply put the food you have introduced on the plate of your child. While it is possible to transform the table into an arena, you must be sure to start with the first step. It is possible to remove the food within a couple of seconds should you have to. If your child does well with the first stage, provide an incentive. The reward can be different, based on what your child is most interested in however the most common suggestions are warm hugs and warm praises. You could also offer small portions of food items that your child likes for example, strawberry ice-cream or a particular game.

As you progress, take additional baby steps such as making your child taste the food, feel the food, move the food closer to the lips, etc. The purpose of these steps is gradually exposing your child's taste buds to food. If you introduce it all at once, it is almost always a recipe for catastrophe. However, you shouldn't give your child ice cream and pizza for the remainder the time. Simple steps such as taking a bite of the food every now and then, or mixing with some other favourite food items, will aid your child in getting used to eating the food.

It is important to recognize that you're not likely be successful on the first go around. If you're a normal mother, you may not be successful for the first couple of times. The most important thing is beginning with baby steps. It is important for your child to be accustomed to the idea of food, regardless of the length of time it takes. If you also encourage your child for each succeeding step, you'll be able to connect the food to positive emotions, which could further aid your cause.

Sleeping

One of the toughest aspects of raising children with autism is getting them to sleep and not wake up. Although other aspects of parenting are difficult and difficult, this takes a particular impact on parents. If your child isn't sleeping and you don't, you'll be too tired to rest. Sleep deprivation can result in an unproductive downward spiral and anxiety. If you're struggling with getting rid of stress and taking good care of yourself, you'll need to refer to the chapter 6 in which we cover seeking help and assistance.

The positive side is that a lot of the advice we've provided in this book can be useful to you. One of the most important is setting up a routine and following it. A routine for bedtime can be beneficial for both you as well as your child. In terms of psychologically it may signal to your body that it's time to stop any activity and recharge. These signals are relaxing for children suffering from ASD or anyone seeking to comprehend everything that that they are receiving from their surroundings.

In order for this to be effective you must establish the routine you'll follow every time. The order of the day isn't as important in the same way as your routine. It is possible to begin with telling your child it's bedtime and then go to the bathroom to brush. Then, the pajamas are put on followed by bedtime stories and finally, it's time to go to bed. It is possible to do it in any order you prefer however, it is essential sticking to the same order each time. It is also possible to create graphs or any other type of visual aid to help your child to remember the precise order of things. As time goes by when your child is familiar with the routine, sleeping is less stress-inducing.

Another tip to consider is to cut down on the amount of rowdy and rough play as the time for bed approaches. When the time for bed comes you child ought to be taking a break from their day's activities and not becoming agitated. While there may be time for fun and play, dependent on your schedule, it shouldn't be a cause for alarming your child. Games like wrestling, tickling or roughhousing are sure to slow down the bedtime. Activities that are more calm, such as drawing or reading a bedtime tale will be the main focus of the time prior to the bedtime.

When you have finally put your child settled The next step in step is to ensure that they are able to sleep peacefully. This involves taking measures like the mummy bag and night light. Children with autism, as well as everyone else are fond of being swaddled and cuddled. Mummy bags have the same effect on children, making it an extremely soothing experience for the children. The nightlights can be a source of the children with a sense of security, particularly when they are scared of dark. A nightlight that has a soft glow can be a source of the comfort. A bright light can make your child sleepy and that's not what you would like to do.

The next tip is self being said, but it's better to be explicit. The comfort of your bed is a necessity. When you're an adult it's difficult to have a comfortable night's sleep in an old and worn-out mattress. In the same way, it's harder for children who have autism to sleep in the same bed. Similar to pillows and sheets.

Toilet training

Toilet training is among the household activities that could reveal how difficult it can be for parents to take care of a child who has autism. Certain children are able to learn to use the toilet at the age of five. However, it may require children with ASD between 9 and 10 years before they are fully toilet-trained. But, because it's a spectrum, certain children are able to master toilet training faster than others. A few tips can help you to train your child faster than without them. Let's look over these tips and discover how you can use each one to train your child.

A crucial step is to set your schedule and time. Toilet training is an extremely involved process, particularly for children suffering from ASD and you have to be prepared to dedicate yourself fully to this process. Changes in health, relocation to a new home, having a baby or any other major change to the family dynamic could affect the process of learning for both of you. Also, you must free yourself from sources that cause stress and pressure. The pressure from family, friends members, or even therapists who are trying to help train your child may cause more stress for you. It's possible that you don't realize it right now that the process of toileting can turn out to be lengthy, and sometimes emotionally-charged process. You don't want to be dealing with all the other issues while you're toilet training.

The following tip works in conjunction with the previous one, and is important to be on the lookout for signs that your kid is ready to go potty training. The age of your child will not affect this determination because children with ASD are prone to developmental issues that make them distinct with normal kids. The indicators to look out for include being clean all night long and asking for a change. When your child begins to be aware of the pain that comes to toilet issues It indicates that they are prepared to use the toilet of a big boy.

When you have determined whether your child's ready to become toilet-trained, you must start filling him up with fluids. Find out the amount of fluids your child is allowed to consume throughout the day with your pediatric physician, and make sure that your child receives the highest amount every day. Mix the water with juice or milk. If your child drinks more fluids than he consumes the more likely it is to vomit. When you are filling your child's bladder with fluids, be sure you have everything you require. It is also possible to bring games or a TV screen for the bathroom. It is important to make your child feel comfortable on your toilet seats. Other options include covering the seat with towels to give it an extra cushion, or buying toilet seats with handles.

To help a child learn to potty it is essential to ensure that your child is sitting on the toilet until magic occurs. It is possible to take short breaks each now and then but your child should be seated at the toilet for as long as they can. In the end, your child may urinate in the toilet. In the event that this occurs, it is important to offer as much praise as you can. Try to demonstrate your pride in your child's accomplishment.

The next step is to concentrate your attention on your child's bowel movements. If your child is for long enough on the toilet it will eventually result in an efficient flow of bowel. In some instances it is possible that your child will be more prone to using diapers to poop than on the toilet. In this situation you'll need to start by determining when your child is most likely to vomit. Let your child go to the bathroom and poop while in the bathroom , as an initial step.

Then, ask him to go to the bathroom and poop using the diaper sitting on the seat of his toilet. Next, proceed to taking his pants off before sitting down on the toilet. And finally, ask him to go to the bathroom without a diaper. The steps could take some time, based on your child's needs and their age, so it's recommended to break them down into smaller steps.

Public spaces

The difficulty of dealing with an autistic child is different when it comes to public areas as you are often required to contend with stares from strangers and explaining the situation to others. The entire situation can be increased when your child decides to have a temper tantrum in a public area such as a restaurant, for instance. The way to handle situations like this will require you to know the child's perspective. Keep in mind that you've established an orderly schedule for him to adhere to. The transition from the routine and moving into a different environment could be extremely stressful the child. At some point you must expect your child to be uncomfortable the new environment. It's just a fact. The focus should not be on what others might think or say, and more on ways to aid your child in adjusting to the new surroundings.

It is not a good idea to feel ashamed of your child unless the remarks and looks actually have a basis. If your child is not being unprofessional, keep your head up. Keep in mind this: your child through extreme discomfort, and anyone who doesn't know what your child goes through can't possibly be able to make a statement or make a contribution.

It is important to know that just like everything else going with your child to public areas is a process of practice, and baby steps. Start at home and imitate some of the behaviors you'll encounter in a restaurant. Inviting your children to the kitchen as you cook. This will provide them with the chance to see food from a different angle generally, and is exactly like what you'll experience at the dining establishment. It's also possible to invite your friends over and create a setting that is as secluded as well as, for want of an appropriate word, noisy as you can. The eatery you choose to go to for a noisy experience, so eating a noisy meal at home isn't appropriate.

For the next step, you should go to areas where there are many people and you will only be spending a few minutes duration there. You can visit the department store or supermarket to purchase some food items. When your child has a good time with the experience and is comfortable, you may take a brief break in a restaurant or cafe. Be aware that the main goal is to get your child familiar with the environment. The trick is that because there are less people in the dining establishment, there's less sensory stimulation for your child , and there is a lower chance of him or her to behave in a way that isn't normal.

After having completed all your practice runs and are confident that you're ready to go on the road It is important to be prepared in case things become out of control. Be aware that your child still a young child and may not behave the way you'd like. It is important to be flexible enough to be able to accept any behavior you witness, and ready to deal with it. In essence, you need an escape route. It is important to determine beforehand how fast you will be able to pay for the cost and take your child to the vehicle.

Chapter 8: Learning & Transitions

One of the biggest concerns that new parents face is what goes through the brain of the toddler? They may seem cute and indifferent to their peers however, after a couple of days, they experience massive changes and eventually become proficient in their language. Even the most experienced parents haven't been capable of coming up with behavior theories. The majority of them do not know how toddlers behave or how they learn from their environment.

Toddlers experience a range of developmental stages during the first stages of their the child's life. They are able to learn by instinct and grow independent much faster than we would anticipate. In most toddlers, communication and, consequently self-expression is an inexplicably important aspect of developing. However, for children that have Autism, communication is a totally different experience. It is essential to pay greater focus on their progress and attempt to be ahead of any noticeable shortcomings.

Based on the time you received an diagnosis from, how much level of attention you pay to each aspect of the social and communicative development process will differ. Toddlers are curious and develop by sharing, playing exploring, and stimulating. Everything they do is infused with meaning. If you can recognize and take care of each stage of their development and development, it could be quite easy to lose sight of time and let this an important stage of their lives slip by.

Play

When a child crawls around and play with his favourite toy, it's a part of a complex learning process that tests those physical rules that govern the world that he is now finding himself. What may appear to be an exercise filled with drool that involves the constant effort to put things into his mouth is really an attempt at understanding the idea of eating and satisfaction.

Toddlers are humans at their most curious and curious stage. Play allows toddlers to discover the answers to a majority of their questions and allows the development of vital survival abilities. As you are aware, children learn to walk through crawling throughout the day before finally moving into walking. Play allows children to acquire experiences, build muscle and learn directly through watching other adults doing it in real time. The toddlers don't have much to do each day other than working on coordination and balance, control of muscles, and endurance. What appears to be play to adults, is actually a challenging and vital mental and physical exercises for development.

Playing with children teaches them about the laws of physics, gravity, pain, and lots more fundamental rules and facts. Play lets toddlers be in contact with various objects and gain knowledge through adapting. Children understand on a certain degree how gravity operates by throwing around toys as well as other items. They learn that when something is raised the same thing will fall down. Play allows them to figure out how the mysterious and new world around them eventually works.

There is a general rule regarding the practice and mastery. It is about the practice of an practice repeatedly until you are able to have mastered the skill you're putting to apply. If an infant is trying to learn to speak the only way that they will ever master the art of talking is to talking in a babbling voice and in short sentences.

Play also helps children develop their imagination. The development of an active imagination is a vital aspect of a child's mental and emotional growth. Their imagination helps them look at the world through another lens and allows their creativity to blossom. Materials such as bricks and Legos are ideal for the child who is imaginative. Making-believe games allow children to discover concepts such as creation and substitution and also improves their fine motor abilities and helping their brains learn.

Sharing can be a complicated aspect of growth. Children tend to pick up on it over time, but some require some encouragement to move to an appropriate direction. As a child grows his brain, it undergoes a variety of changes. At some stage, he'll be able to comprehend complex emotional cues from watching the parents and caregivers around time. Sharing is a process that can be learned and learned over the passage of time. A child in preschool is likely to be more knowledgeable about sharing than a typical toddler. Children are naturally self-centered and self-serving. They don't appreciate the benefits of sharing.

However, just like the language, and various other complicated social and interaction actions sharing is an essential life skill that helps you to build and keep relationships with others. Sharing is a way to bring people together and teach people a bit about turning over, sacrifice, and dealing with disappointments.

Sharing is an essential social and survival skill, it is crucial to observe your child's progress and their interactions. Many children have a difficult to share, which is why it is crucial to educate your child to share in a safe and non-threatening manner. The most effective way to educate your child to share is to make it clear that this was his choice right from the beginning. For instance, if, for example, you discuss an acquaintance of your child's, and how he played with his toys with the class Your child will be enticed to emulate him. This strategy is particularly useful for preschoolers and others who are of school age. It is also advisable to be practicing sharing food and toys with your child, and then encourage him whenever he manages to do it correctly. It is crucial to help your child realize when he's performing something wrong or correct. Beliefs and actions should be monitored at all times, particularly for children who are just getting introduced to the social norms and habits.

Sharing exercises with your children is an enjoyable way to teach the child about turning and expressing dissatisfaction. In a moment, depriving a child toys or any other kind of reward will help the child to handle disappointment, and also teach him about patience. While sharing is highly encouraged among children in their early years however, clear boundaries must be set. Certain things must be kept from sharing. On the basic level, each child is a bonder to things like clothes or toys, and eventually, they are inseparable from the item. These items should not be utilized in normal games of sharing.

Children aren't all accustomed to the idea of sharing. They don't assume that it's necessary or beneficial. In cases of extreme occurrences like these it is recommended to introduce some form of punishment to help them straighten out. Implementing a moderate punishment system can help them more easily adapt and understand the idea of sharing. If they don't share, you should inform them the reason they're being punished and remove the toy for a specified amount of time. Naturally, you shouldn't penalize children who don't behave in similarly. The toddlers don't view sharing the same way that preschoolers and school students do.

They think you're penalizing them every when you remove their toys. Therefore, whether you're sharing your toys with them or scolding them for doing it they'll generally react in similarly. Retribution won't fix any issue. They're not emotionally capable of learning something from punishment.

Preschoolers, on one they can empathize on an extent. They comprehend the concept of fairness, and they see the rationale when you give someone else the chance to play with the toy they enjoy. The punishment of removing the toy they have and explaining the reasons behind the type of punishment you're imposing is more appealing to pre-schoolers. Although they can be impatient, they are able to comprehend cause and effect on a certain degree as well. They are also more likely be correct by the method you choose to use for punishment.

Students who attend school are more mature and more likely to be able to appreciate sharing and the lessons in the punishment you pick. They are also easier to think about and communicate concepts to. Their minds are like sponges that absorb the important lessons you consider important.

Letting your toddler play

The act of watching your child's play is a simple method to monitor the progress of your child and making adjustments to his intellectual and social development. The majority of new parents do not be aware of this, but it is what they do the majority times when they're doing nothing but feeding their children or tidying after their children.

As an adult, you could like taking your children under your care and watching the development of their children. However, occasionally it's best to let them explore and play in the world on their own. The world is big and frightening but what's truly terrifying would be letting children grow self-sufficient.

Children by nature are incredibly dependent upon their families. They rely upon them to provide food, fun and even to play. Let your child play in the absence of the presence of you will help them to be more independent and discover the world around them. As time passes, they'll be able to accept that you won't always be available to watch children play and will rely on you less.

When children spend time with their older counterparts too often they can be stifled in their imagination and creativity. If a child is left with nothing more than toys to play with, he is left with no option to think up complex stories and adventures for himself. Adults usually do the majority of the imaginative thinking during the playgroups with children. When play is led by children the mind wanders and they create amazing creatures, beings and animals.

It aids in building confidence and social autonomy. Children who are allowed to themselves to explore and grow over time are more likely to develop a greater awareness of their own self. They will have a better chance of being comfortable in a variety of social situations and be able to interact with others who are their age easily.

Self-led play can teach children to relax and become more peaceful.

Different developmental and cognitive stages for children

A Swiss psychologist who was a developmentalist named Jean Piaget posited that there are four distinct cognitive development phases in the development of a child. The classification was first proposed in 1936. Although there has been a change since the time the work of Jean Piaget is highly regarded and is considered an established benchmark. Some other great psychologists have come up with an almost complete division of a child's cognitive development. The division they propose can account for the times that Piaget's classification mixed up. The more recent classifications aren't able to go deep as Piaget's. So, we'll look at the two theories that are popular.

Piaget's theory tries to explain the cognitive processes of children and answer the age-old question "What happens in the mind of a child?" According to his theory, the development of cognition begins at the time the child is born, and continues until the age of 15 or so years old. At that point, the child begins to think as an adult. As the years, he gets more proficient and skilled at it. The initial stage is the sensorimotor phase, which is followed by concrete, preoperational as well as formal stage. We have already covered the various phases of development in the first chapter under the development of your infant. The following picture is more detailed and describes the specific changes that take place within your child's brain. It's worth reiterating.

Sensorimotor development is the initial phase of a child's cognitive development. It starts as soon as the baby is born and continues until about two years old. At this point children are able to perceive reality through interaction with the world along with other stimuli. At this point the process of learning is swift and repetitious, and is done through assimilation as well as accommodation. The child engages with the world through the senses. At this point it's crucial that the child identifies his own reality and creates an individual self which is separate from his surroundings.

The child also attempts to give the significance of objects at this phase. The child isn't quite in the right place intellectually and must rely on actual things and situations to comprehend the various thoughts. This is when children begin to form relationships with objects and toys and are unable to share and empathizing. They interpret concepts and thoughts in a literal way and struggle with abstract ideas. The preoperational stage usually is about 5 years old. It is typically between the ages of 2-7.

The third stage is known as the functional stage that is concrete. It generally runs from years 7 to 11, and during this period the child is beginning to think in a complex manner and try to answer the questions that he's always asked. They begin to generalize and depend on logic to understand particular things. They begin to understand concepts such as transformations, and then they develop the capacity to be emotionally receptive and understanding. At this point they are still struggling with the concept of abstraction. They're still very literal and only comprehend concrete and solid things.

It is the most important phase of a child's cognitive development. At this point they begin to formulate hypotheses and comprehend the abstract. Then they begin thinking more morally ethically, philosophically and politically. They start to think more inductively and use general information to form their own opinions. They are basically miniature adults who form themselves with their ideas and views about how the world is.

The second class is focused more on the mental aspects of development in children and instead, focuses on development in general. It concentrates on the social, cognitive physical, and social development of each child, and meticulously records the changes that occur over the course of. The classification breaks down the child's development into five distinct phases. These are infant, newborn Toddler, Preschool and school-age. The infant stage lasts approximately one month. The baby's movements and reactions are usually automated. For instance, babies cry when they are in need of something and want to be held and taken care for.

The infant stage begins immediately following the newborn stage and continues until the beginning one year into existence. The new stage of infanthood comes with a rapid growth in skills and bodily control as well as strength and mobility. That means that your child must begin picking up things and crawling about as well as moving his hands and sitting up without assistance.

The third stage is known as the toddler stage. It usually occurs between the age of 1-3 and in this period you'll notice your child is walking , climbing and jumping, drawing, and sometimes stacking. The development of language is significant at this point and your child should be able communicate with tiny phrases. Also, it is during this stage that your child must be assessed for autism or other illness.

The preschool stage runs from ages 3-5. This is when the majority of children begin to develop their motor abilities. They develop independence and are able to dress themselves. They also have greater body strength and can leap or draw, jump and stand on one leg for several seconds.

This is known as the school-age stage , which lasts about six years , beginning at six to twelve years old. In this time, they grow more independent, responsible and confident. They also become more social. They begin to make lasting relationships and acquire sexual preferences and characteristics.

The process of raising a child isn't an easy job. Sometimes, you have to look back and allow them to develop into the person you think they are. For children with autism, the stages of development are generally identical. They grow physically, cognitively and emotionally just as their peers. They require a little assistance in the social and communication aspects of their development. As parents, you have the responsibility to bridge this gap and aid them to integrate into society.

Chapter 9: Your Child And Your Family

Autism can do much more than devastate your savings and financial resources and also stress relationships with partner or spouse. It could affect nearly all members of your family in either way. A single family member could cause you to be insensitive for the demands of others in your family. In the blink of an eye, children who require assistance receive little or none even if they need help. You're captivated by the health of one child. siblings and brothers feel that they are less important or have less. If you don't take care the needs of children will grow and develop into an intense hatred which will result in them blaming the other brother or you. The present chapter we'll be looking at ways to stop this from taking place.

The focus will be on the suffering of your siblings, your brother sister, mother and in general, every member of your family. The needs of your children are equally important so this section will make sure that you don't forget to consider your children while taking care of your child.

Care for your partner

Parents who don't have partners who they can share parenting with. If you're one of the fortunate few that have someone to rely on it is important to appreciate that you're blessed to not be on this journey by yourself.

No matter if you're married or not the spouse you have is your co-pilot and they are a part of your life to help ease the immense stress that raising an autistic child could cause. It's not a secret that children are blessed regardless of the condition they're born with however, they can also be difficult sometimes. It is important to acknowledge this and take advantage of the advantages of having an individual who makes your journey much more enjoyable. This means you need to find time in your busy schedule to attend to the needs of your loved ones too.

They may have needs that are physical or emotional. However, as you are in your ability to do something to address it, you must. You may need to take a break for a day or warm meal or may need to discuss your child's health and the changes that you are both facing.

As a great friend do not focus on only clear calls for assistance. Find out what they require even if they do not say anything. Do things to keep the romance alive in your relationship , and then seek out what they're feeling without having them inquire. You were in an intimate relationship before children were born There is no reason to believe that this has to change due to the fact that there is a kid who has special needs. It is important to be the same person you've always been regardless of what happens.

Take charge of the other kids

The other children might not show it however they are dependent on you as much as their sister or brother who has autism. They may not be able to tell you because they're unable to communicate the issue in words, however not listening to their needs is among the most costly mistakes you could make. Children aren't as innovative or sensitive as adults. They can feel secluded and jealous when someone in the world is the focus of attention at all times.

It is important to take care of their needs as well. It is normal that you may not be able spend time with them the same way as you do with your child who has special needs However, you can keep anger and other negative emotions from forming by teaching them the importance of commitment and sacrifice.

Introduce the idea that autism is a problem to your children and make them realize why you need to look after their sister or brother. It is also important to help them talk about autism with you. It is common for kids across the globe with siblings who are autistic. The discussion about autism can show them that they're not lonely as they may think and help them to understand the differences between their siblings and their parents are.

A little one-on-one time with them in the distraction of their sibling is a wonderful option to attend to their requirements. Attention cannot be substituted by gifts. Plan fun outings or trips with your friends and make an effort to get to know them outside of the home.

They can also be put in charge of their siblings. In many families that have siblings, the sibling who does not suffer from a communication disorder is entrusted with their needs for the sibling with the disorder. This is an excellent approach to help them become used to the responsibility and strengthen the bond between siblings. Teach them the importance of protecting your brother and show them that you appreciate the sacrifices they make.

Also, don't offend them by minimizing their struggles or refusing look at their side of an disagreement. If there are arguments among siblings, as they do in the normal course and they do, don't choose to side with their autistic sibling. Bring a bit of equality by not being able to trust your opinions. If they face a challenge that appears insignificant do not dismiss them completely. It is important to acknowledge their discomfort. It could be a cry to be heard. By ignoring it, they believe that you are not as fond of them.

Be focused on each and every family member in your nuclear as well as extended family

The requirements of your parents, grandparents, cousins aunts, uncles acquaintances, and the rest of your family may not be as important as those for your husband, children suffering from ASD or siblings. However, these needs should not be overlooked. Friends and family members can be your backup when your resources and strength have fallen short. If you care for your family and include them in the daily routine of your daily life they can be beneficial and ease the burden of raising your whole family without any external help.

If you establish your bond sufficiently, they may be a potential babysitters, investors, support groups, or even helpers. With their help the child's journey will be filled with family members and family members who cherish your child as much as you do.

The best method to develop relationships with them is to help them when they truly need help and assisting them in every ways you are able to. Hosting family meals and inviting them to attend. Go to social gatherings which you consider significant to them. Spend time with them and talk to them. one-on-one time with them. Be kind to them just as your own child or sibling. Don't be afraid to speak about your hopes and fears of your children. If you're able to talk with your child about their family members, whom can you talk with about it?

Chapter 10: Looking All My Ways Of

Communicating

Communication methods can be different among children who have autism. They develop their own ways of communicating based on their abilities. In general, hand gestures, eye contact and expressions on the face are effective ways to communicate with children.

Each child with autism will possess a distinct intellectual and social development. The development of that child determines the way in which he or she is communicating with other people. Some children aren't able to use language or speak in any way. Some may possess the ability to speak with a bit or complete ability. A lot of kids have difficulty making vocal sounds and aligning body language to their vocabulary.

Therefore, it's clear that generalization isn't helpful in understanding an autistic child. However, specific classifications will assist you in learning the patterns of communication of an individual.

Language is rigid or repetitive.

If the child is gifted with speaking abilities, it's possible the child exhibits an inflexibility and repetition when speaking. They may say the same phrases over and over repeatedly during conversations. The act of counting numbers is among the daily activities observed in these children. When a child hears an interesting word, he or could repeat it repeatedly and repeatedly.

It is also typical for those with Autism to talk loudly or use a distinct tone while speaking. A robotic voice or speech that has a tone of singing can be a possibility too.

Uneven language skills

If a child does develop speech, might have a problem with the language. Normal language skills don't often happen in these children. Their vocabulary may be exceptional in particular areas that fall within their area of interest.

However, it can be difficult for them to construct sentences using those words like the typical child would. Some children are unable to understand the meaning behind the words they have read or hear. This is why their reaction time is generally slower than that of others. This is the reason why many teachers and parents make the mistake of believing that the child is hearing impaired.

Extraordinary talent

A child with autism's brain explores different ways of communicating. This is the reason why they develop extraordinary skills in a variety of cases. The talent is based on the needs and interests of the youngster. Some begin playing the piano from an early age, and others grow to be exceptional at maths, memorizing, or history. But, these skills do not guarantee a certain level of proficiency. A lot of children simply select a method that allows them to talk to their surroundings.

Limited nonverbal communication

Gesture-based language is a challenge for children. Autism is a condition that makes it difficult for children to comprehend the significance behind the gesture of a finger towards an object. Eye contact can be difficult for these children. The behavior can leave others question their fascination. If the child is interested in what you're speaking, he or she may not be looking at you with straight eyes.

Insufficient the ability to communicate non-verbally generally leads to inappropriate behaviors and an aggressive personality. The child has no means to express his or her anger.

Social interactions are difficult in the traditional way.

The ability to comprehend the viewpoint of others is a challenge for children of this age. They typically interpret the meaning of what you tell them or say to them. This limitation is apparent when a child is reading, watching films, or interacts with others in the world. The unique thoughts or inter-personal motivations of people around them can be difficult to comprehend for an autistic child. They are unable to comprehend the idea or idea simply by looking at the behaviour of others.

The ability to concentrate on one topic is also a challenge for children who have autism. They are usually immersed in their thoughts and thoughts, as well as the words they find themselves drawn to. This can affect their ability to engage in conversations with other people. However, if they are presented with a subject that interests them, they could talk for hours and give lengthy monologues. However, this could impact negatively in a variety of situations. For instance, a child cannot be a part of a debate when others are required to speak about the same subject.

A child with autism typically doesn't display the social judgement that they feel. This means that the child could start uttering phrases or words in public without thinking about what others would view them. This can also impact the child's ability to comprehend the importance of facts. The child may be a bit uninformed in a social context. They don't know the hurt of others because they believe that they are speaking the truth.

Autism-related children aren't aware of the concept of changing the style of conversation to suit the other person in the conversation. As an example, they speak to their teachers in the same way they interact with their peers. Therefore their words and tone can be considered rude to a lot of people. Most of the time the child will use the TV character of his choice to express himself. The child may play the TV character while interacting in real everyday.

Autistic children may possess the ability to lie. However, they don't use lies to trick or fool other people. The child might lie to avoid the person who he dislikes.

A remarkable ability to search for deep knowledge makes these children difficult to talk to. The majority of the time children will choose their most interesting fact during the conversation, and then begin talking over and over about the aspect. This is why a point occurs where the discussion turns dull.

The brain of children is always looking for patterns of communication. These children continue to store the behavior, words, as well as strategies in their brain. Sometimes, they use older patterns in their interactions with others. It could include an aggressive approach to express anger or anger, self-abuse, pacing as well as other undesirable behaviors. Teachers and parents can help the child learn the best techniques to utilize communication patterns.

The Visual Method of Thinking

Autism-related children use visuals as their primary language. In actuality, all spoken and written words are able to take shape in the brain of autistic children. This could be a distinct advantage for the child when it is able to motivate them to the right way.

Every child has their own unique imagining technique for creating pictures and sound for words. Some use sound and music to help them understand difficult subjects like math.

Visual thinking is beneficial in many ways for children with autism. For instance, Temple Grandin, who is a well-known scientist and engineer is autistic and is a visual thinker.

In the majority of children diagnosed with autism, a visual-based method of learning is the most effective. This helps overcome the issue of language and verbal barriers and helps the child be able to comprehend ideas, emotions and information quickly. Visual thinking is a great tool to enhance social interaction and to teach various skills to children. Pictures, and symbols can aid children with autism understand math more effectively than formulas written. Therefore, instead in the words "wash your face" on the bathroom's door it is better to put up an image of the child taking care of his facial. This will aid your child in understanding and remember the job. Many of the daily tasks are more comfortable for children by teaching them the right method. Sorting laundry, folding clothes and many other methods are easily taught to your child. All you need to do is place visually-based reminders into the appropriate areas or present them to your child in the appropriate time.

Here are some suggestions for teachers and parents to include target visual thinking in teaching children who are young and have autism:

Make A visible structure

The concentration levels differ for children suffering from this disorder. Therefore, it is important to develop a plan that is comfortable for your child. If you are looking to instruct children on everyday activities or introduce a new idea, you should decide on the time frame. This is the time when you may take a little part of the idea and translate it into pictures.

Utilizing the visual aspect of learning

Images, picture cards line drawings, and many other objects are great for tapping into the aspect of visual learning for the child. It is possible to use stickers in your daily routine of your child. Separate different sets of visuals into distinct sections of the routine and create a safe and comfortable setting to ensure that the child is able to quickly absorb the lessons.

Use communication devices

A communication device is a fun method of learning. You can pick the portable device that has colorful illustrations and signs. After that, you can encourage your child to use the appropriate keys to speak. This will help gradually to improve the skills of speaking.

Assistance with social interactions

Parents want to see the satisfaction of their children. As early as a child the joy of a child is having fun and making friends with other people. This task is extremely difficult for parents with children who is autistic. The lack of connection caused by communication difficulties can make it difficult for the child to communicate with other people. If the child does attempt to communicate, he / is usually wrongly interpreted.

But, it is feasible to assist an autistic child develop their social interactive abilities.

Teachers and parents can put different strategies to guide children to take steps in the right direction for social interaction.

Method 1: Explain social interactions using an example

As we mentioned, children make use of their environment to establish a pattern for interaction. This means that you can apply the same approach when presenting social interactions as models. However, this isn't something that can be done once. You must constantly develop unique and innovative models to assist your child to improve their social skills. You must explain every aspect of every social skill you wish to teach the child. Additionally, explain the emotional motivations and values of these social interactions in the form of words. This will assist in understanding non-verbal interactions.

It is possible to make your own list of scenarios that are social and spend some time explain each one to your child. This method is the most effective when you are able to explain the scenario immediately after the incident happens. If you witness a social situation in a public area it is possible to quickly explain the reasons and consequences of the incident. Talk to your child about expressions of facial expressions, words and other actions using facts.

Be sure to remember that explaining is essential in trying to enhance social skills in children who has autism. Your task is to translate the non-verbal aspects of interaction into descriptions of verbal interactions.

Method 2: Make use of the imitation of a role or role-play

Children may find it difficult to switch the vocabulary or tone of voice to convey the correct messages. It is possible to help them get more adept at speaking and writing through role-playing. For example parents can behave as a rule and request your child to reply to questions. You can also play the roles of different individuals who are before your child regular basis. Regular practice will enable the child to comprehend the proper usage of words and voice tone while talking to others.

Making up scenarios that are hypothetical creates an environment for communication within the child. This method helps to navigate through conversations when the child has to deal with social situations in his real life. You can train your child to speak with the correct manner and change the speed of speech, and allow time to allow people to comprehend sentences.

Method 3: Gather videos in a set

Children with autism learn to imitate and mimic what they see in films or television programs. It is possible to use this as teach advantage. A set of videos that demonstrate all the desirable behaviors can benefit the child. You can play these videos frequently and discuss the details of the current behavior. It will become easier for your child to learn the lessons and implement the same principles in different situations.

Because videos can be used to create visual memories, they remain in the brain of the child for a long period of time. They store the details of words and gestures in their minds and try to imitate the way they behave. Regular practice using videos is a good idea to increase the social skills of youngsters.

Approach 4: Utilize the most recent technology in everyday life

Technology has advanced significantly and has made significant advances in mobile communication. There are numerous options and methods to improve the speech of children with autism. Numerous apps can help children to tackle their speech problems. Mobile phone technology to transform words into sounds or symbols. This makes communication more secure and efficient for children.

When working with speech, it's important to determine whether the child has any other problems in addition to autism. Vision, motor issues and other issues can hinder the ability of a child to speak. Find technologies that are compatible with the needs of the child.

Method 5: Have a fun game

An enjoyable activity is atypical for any child, no matter any illness or condition. Simple games can aid in encouraging positive social behaviours among children who are autistic. It is possible to teach your child to comprehend facial signals and behave in accordance with guidelines of your game. Repetition of the same actions during a game of fun will aid in learning those facial expressions as well as their meaning. Your child will begin to recognize non-verbal signals when you pick the right game.

It is essential to pick games that are focused on specific concepts and skills that you wish to impart to your child. The ability to guess movies using non-verbal gestures will enhance the social skills that the kid. You can also choose several other games according to the child's level of interest. Make it enjoyable to use it for good.

Approach 6: Take your pet home

The research suggests that pets assist children with autism to develop social abilities. Pets help children to bond to an emotional level and form bonds. This same skill can be helpful when the child is in public. For instance, the emotional bond with a pet may help the child more open to asking questions. They feel more confident in asking questions.

Pets can also be a good conversation starter with children. Children can share the stories of their pets and share experiences to other kids. So, the other children find it more enjoyable to talk to the child. This increases confidence in social interactions.

Approach 7 The child should be the one in charge

The mere imitation and practice of not enough. The child needs to be exposed to situations in the social realm and be in charge of the situation. You must take your child to secure but authentic social situations to allow them to utilize their abilities. For example, a games event at your home is a safe place that allows your child to have fun with other kids as well as parents. The kid can have fun with friends and utilize the skills you've been teaching them for some time.

Let them be for a time to allow them to enhance their interaction. However, you must be alert to stop the action if it could get out of control. This strategy is definitely somewhat uncertain, but you need to believe in the child and let them attempt it again and again in order to develop better social abilities.

Method 8: Reward good behaviour

Just like any other child that is autistic, children are also motivated by being given rewards for their actions. Teachers and parents typically observe their behavior and how they interact with pets, peers and other individuals.

If you notice an improvement in the child's behavior Show your appreciation by rewarding your child. This can help reinforce the positive behavior the child is displaying. Even small rewards such as the toy they love most or meal, or even a trip to a place that they love can have a significant impact. They act as a way to reinforce and encourage children to display the same behavior frequently.

Approach 9: Provide interactions that are in line with child's desires

If someone shares similar interests to ours It makes it easier for friendships to grow stronger. Even strangers can be close while drinking coffee and discussing their favourite sport or music, or even their favorite hobby. This is also true for children who have autism. If you set them up in a setting that includes others who share similar interests and hobbies this can increase their social interactions. A chess or dance class, art class and other relevant settings can create social interactions that are enjoyable and beneficial for your child. Be sure that children in the class are the same age range like your son or daughter. So, your child will be able to develop behavior that is suitable for their age.

It is possible to use a simple combination of strategies from all the ones mentioned. But, it's important to be persistent and maintain patience. Change won't come over the course of a single day. Furthermore, the effort you put into it today will benefit your child's future. Follow a step-by-step method to make social interactions enjoyable for your child. Begin with introducing the abilities, where you will explain how these social skills are used. Next, you can move on to conversations, such as vocal tone and vocabulary. Then, you can attempt to make them more effective in various social situations.

Find out what places and things Scare Me the Most

Fear is a very common issue that can be found in autism children. Knowing what places and things can assist you in managing the child's behavior successfully.

The fear of mechanical objects

Many machines can trigger fear or phobias in children who have autism. For example children may be scared of ceiling fans or hair dryers. In the same way, many children struggle to remain in the vicinity of blenders and vacuum cleaners, washing machines as well as other mechanical objects which produce constant sound. For some children, this fear may become more extreme when they begin to feel scared of things like clothing, can openers and other items that are mechanical.

Fear of the heights

While the fear of heights is prevalent for many, children with autism do not know the best way to communicate their fears. Therefore, they behave in a bizarre manner that can hurt themselves or others in certain circumstances. Things like elevators and escalators and many other high places can trigger anxiety, and can trigger anger and aggression.

Fear of going to certain places

The presence of small spaces or crowds can make children feel uncomfortable. For many, the discomfort can reach a point of anxiety. Therefore, it's possible for children to be able to resist entering the tiny bathroom or bedrooms.

In contrast, certain youngsters develop a fear of large open spaces. If the space is too big, like an athletic stadium the children may feel anxious to the point that they are unable to leave.

If a child with autism experiences a negative incident that was related to a specific location, it could trigger an intense sense of discontent regarding the location within their mind. For instance, if we speak about poor services or dirty bathrooms at restaurant, your child might be prone to fear the restaurant in question.

Some children also fear being locked in a room, and some get anxious in a space with the doors left open. This is because of the experiences children experience in their everyday life. Autism is a condition that affects his or her methods to perceive the environment. This causes a range of bizarre anxieties about places within the brain that the person with autism.

The fear of the weather

The weather can be a bad information for everyone. However, it could be an absolute disaster for children who have autism. If the child has reached an age where they are able to, the weather could appear like a storm. A storm could appear like a doomsday scenario to young children.

Fear of catastrophes

The thought of unwelcome events comes to everyone's mind. But, a normal person is able to separate those thoughts and remain sane. Autism sufferers don't have these abilities. They actually take their anxieties to the next degree and put it into a tangible within their minds.

In an automobile, a child may feel confident about the incident. Similar to that, children can be terrified of drowning around the water. Infection by bacteria is another major anxiety that children develop in the course of time. But, even at a young age, they may have fears of losing their toys or being injured while playing.

Things you must avoid in the case of the fear of an autistic child.

If a child's fear, parents and teachers typically make a few errors.

* Not recognizing fear

For the average person, fear can be defined as beating heart, fast-paced breathing as well as crying, hiding, sweating and many other symptoms. But a child who has autism does not use these typical methods of expressing the fear. Fear is for them an emotion that is complex and communicating the emotion is more difficult than. They might use shouting to express the fear. It is possible to think that they are not listening to your voice or yelling at you in a rude manner. Children often stop doing things and remain still when they fear something.

The root of fear is as similar to an autistic child just like any human being. Everyone wants to be safe and avoid being afraid. But an autistic child may not always have a clear way to express their anxiety. Moving clothes and aggression, asking the same question repeatedly, as well as other indicators could be the reactions.

For many children, fear can have an impact on their digestion. It occurs when a child begins to tighten the throat because of anxiety. This can hinder eating and digestion slows down. These signs could result in breakdowns. It is therefore important to address it before it gets any worse.

* Never anticipating fear

Another mistake teachers and parents do is to not anticipate the anxiety. The child may begin feeling anxious in ordinary settings like a shopping mall or in a class. Fear of songs that are sudden or eating a brand new kind of food or other could be a possibility. These kinds of situations are so common that we tend to ignore these situations. Yet an autistic child may be afraid of situations that normally make other children smile.

The one thing you don't want is to be shocked by an unexpected reaction. The best way to avoid this is to know the things that are new or unique within the surroundings that might cause the child to be fearful.

* Not acknowledging the fear.

Certain words make you ignorant and unreliable towards children with autism. Parents and teachers often are prone to saying or thinking these things:

* No need to be worried

* Fear of things that are harmless

* They're not scary.

What you should know is that nobody gets scared for no justification. Fear is about the things that scare them, not necessarily about things that do not cause you to be scared. Things and events that are familiar may be extremely difficult, overwhelming and unpredictably for the autistic kid. They are unable to determine the root cause or the effect of an issue, and it can lead to anxiety.

In general, children are taught to be cautious from particular dangers, such as dogs, heights, moving vehicles, and so on. Therefore, the presence of these scenarios fills children's minds with all kinds of terrifying thoughts. It's the same for children with autism when they look at something that's frightening for them. The reasons behind the fears of autistic children aren't frequent, it isn't possible to ignore the causes of their fears.

Children with autism are scared because of misinterpretations by teachers and parents. The impact of anxiety on your child simply by acknowledging and accepting the fear. Your help can create the child with a sense of security and ease anxiety and anxiety.

Chapter 11: What Is The Best Way To Be Able

To Identify And Handle My Breakdowns

Beyond the general fear an autistic child may even reach a point of devastation. A meltdown or breakdown is where the child loses ability to control the actions of others.

A breakdown occurs when a child is overwhelmed by certain objects or places or events. The brain's sensory system is overstimulated and can lead to uncontrolled behavior. It is caused by the combination of child's fear of the world and outdoor simulations.

Recognizing indicators that could result in problems

Most often, a temper tantrum causes a decline for children with autism. If the child isn't allowed something they desire it can lead to an outburst and eventually the breaking point. Similar to a desire receive attention, being denied access to things they love or toys, and many other factors can trigger tantrums.

Therefore, you must discover the stimuli that cause breakdowns. Examine the fear-based feelings within the everyday activities of your child. Make notes of the things that act to stimulate breakdowns. A checklist will aid in identifying the needs desires, items you do not want as well as situations and locations.

Resolving problems

Take a break to relax

If you are able to spot the first indications of breakdowns before they become serious enough the technique could be effective. Children can shift their focus to something that's amusing for them. Being happy can aid in preventing breakdowns before they begin. You can play your favorite tune for your child, make smiles, or even give toys that aid in changing the mood of your child.

Make sure your child is away from objects that could be dangerous for them.

When an autistic child suffers difficulties, any dangerous objects could be dangerous. It is crucial that you keep glass items as well as other hazardous items out of reach your child. Create a space that is large open spaces to ensure that your child does not be injured in the event of a meltdown. It is essential that you remain close to your child as separation can cause a sense of terror.

Provide a sense that you are secure

If your child is at the point of breakdown then you must make sure that the child is in a safe place for them to be peaceful. Begin by eliminating any triggers that could cause anxiety. If you're driving in a car or even at home, be sure that you turn off the music.

If the accident occurs in a public area take a break and locate an enjoyable and peaceful area. Peace and tranquility can lessen the impact of a break-down.

It's true that not all places allow you to create a tranquil atmosphere. Therefore, it is important to make use of your arms and hold the child in order to create an impression of security. It may take some effort and effort however, you will be successful in calming your child.

Make sure you invest in items for sensory management

The experts suggest that you keep your kit filled with items that will help you in case of breakdowns. A kit will help in the event of a meltdown occurring in a public place.

Here are the essentials you'll need to have in your kit

* Headphones with noise cancellation capacity

* Blanket with weighted

* Sunglasses

* Food items that are crunchy

* Children's most-loved scent lotion for hands

* Hand wipes

* The child's most loved toy

Sunglasses are a great way to protect your child from the harmful light sources. When they go out, children are exposed to bright light and fixtures that produce fluorescent hues. The lights can create feelings of terror. Therefore, it is recommended to wear sunglasses that lower the harshness and brightness of the lights.

A blanket made of soft fabric and weight could provide gentle pressure on your child's body. In the event of a breakdown the pressure acts as a positive stimuli and helps reduce the stress. Keep the cover in your kit for emergencies all the time.

It is also a reason for hunger that can cause breakdowns, and therefore snacks could be a great option to have in your bag. It is recommended to choose a hard or chewy snack that can let your child concentrate on oral activities.

Outside noises are among the top triggers that increase the likelihood of breakdowns. So, it is recommended to purchase high-end headphones for your child. Be sure that the headphones stop outside noise. This can help manage the child's behavior when in loud public spaces.

A lot of children who have this issue exhibit sensitivity to smell and even touch. Hand wipes and lotion can help you manage your child's behavior and prevent from problems. If your child accidentally touches an object they don't want to it is possible to immediately use hand wipes to ease his or her irritation . You can also offer the preferred lotion to ensure that your hands smell exactly like the scent that he prefers.

Be cool and stay cool

It is impossible to help your child who is having a breakdown If you are intimidated or scared. Make sure you remain cool in these circumstances. It can be difficult due to the sudden aggression that the kid displays. However, if you are unable to react to the child's moves, it may increase the violence of the child. Be quiet and speak at a slower pace. Do not attempt any forceful actions to intimidate the child.

Monitor child's diet

The chemical reactions of food items could be a cause for breakdowns. For example, too much sugar can increase the enthusiasm of a child, making them susceptible to breakdowns. Consuming too much carbohydrates can also cause anxiety and cause breakdowns in children who are autistic.

Your job is to watch the diet of your child. Try to make their diet as gluten-free as possible, or cut down on sugar and carbs in meals.

Beware of sudden movements or actions

When your child is in the beginning stages of a breakdown, it isn't possible to do any abrupt actions. Hugging hands, holding hands or other actions require explanation before they can be done. In the absence of explanation, children may be scared and can trigger a meltdown. Always be sure to inform your child or parents before making a make any changes.

Breakdowns can be one of the most challenging aspects of autism, for parents and children. As a result of sensory stimulation children aren't able to feel they have any control over their behavior. Therefore, teachers, parents and other people involved in the process are held accountable for the wellbeing of children. Your behavior determines how serious an injury can be for your child. This is why it is important prepare yourself using these tips.

Help Me to Understand What You Want

Because communication is a key problem in autism, it can take many hours to communicate with the children with autism and get across your message. A simple inquiry about what they like to eat is often difficult to find an answer to. However, these issues shouldn't hinder you from looking after your child.

Be ready to discuss

It's easy to stay clear of all contact with children who are autistic. But, it could make children feel alone and isolated from the rest of the world. It is important to build an interest in connecting with your child. Your effort can help your child become more open as they grow older.

Autism is a condition that causes children to be autistic. isn't able to talk because they aren't eager to speak. It's because they don't be able to comprehend what you're saying. Therefore, it is best to not take it personally and be more understanding and patient with the child. This is the most important step to help you have a positive conversation and communicate your message to your child.

Utilize their interests to express your ideas

It's impossible to make an autistic child discuss things they don't like. The best strategy is to leverage their curiosity in your favor. You can shape a conversation into topics they are interested in and then alter the topic according to the questions you'd like to inquire about. This can help you avoid being shut down by the child.

As you've probably guessed that children with autism like to debate topics that are interesting to them. They may be boring for you. However, ensure that you convey the impression that you are interested in the discussion. Make use of words to convey your enthusiasm and convey your message that is hidden within the sentences.

Select the appropriate moment to discuss

It is also a crucial element when you are trying to talk with an autistic child. A majority of kids who suffer from ASD tend to adhere to an established timetable. If you interrupt them or attempt to alter the schedule with your speech this can cause issues. Your child may not pay attention to you completely and just do their own thing.

It is essential to determine the state of mind of a child at that moment. If the child is constantly contemplating something, or if the child is focused on other things. These factors are important if prefer to pick an time that the child is at peace. That way, you'll be given full focus.

Make sure to be truthful and simple.

Autism does not allow children to comprehend the meaning of our words, metaphors and other abstract terms. It's impossible for your message to be communicated if your words don't make sense to them. Avoid any metaphorical or abstract speech that demands the ability to comprehend the hidden emotions.

Make sure to use facts and make your sentences simple. So, you can send a clear message your child and ensure the conversational flow.

Monitor non-verbal signs

Autism children develop distinctive behaviors that help them communicate their message. They can be different between children and that's why it is important to learn about these behaviors first. Keep in mind the signals you receive when engaging in conversations. A hand gesture, an action or similar sentences and other indicators can tell you if your child is at ease speaking to your or.

Make use of sound and visual together

Combining visual cues and your voice can enhance the quality of conversations. If the child can read, write down the words you would like to use. Then, you can show the sentence to your child, and repeat that sentence. You can ask your child to write down the answer or read it aloud. You can also use other visual aids in order to convey your message and have a successful conversations with the child.

For children who aren't able to write or read, pictures can be a great visual aid. For example, you could draw an apple, and say"apple" and then say "apple." Then, ask if the child would like an apple. If you provide a range of choices then the child could choose one of his preferred choices. It could require some time and repetition for the child to become used to these activities.

Make your sentences descriptive

When you are giving instructions to your child, try to make it as clear as you possibly can. For instance, instead saying, "It's dinner time."

162

Speak, "You should go wash your hands, then sit down at the dining table to enjoy your dinner."

In the same way, if you're making a gesture towards an object or space you can mention the name of the object and then the desired action from your child. This will allow the child to perform what you wish.

Fewer questions, more statements

If you ask "How do you feel?" The child may begin to think about what he or she is feeling at the moment. Autistic children take their questions carefully and want to give the perfect answer. In the pursuit of perfection, they often do not answer in any way. Certain questions cause them to feel trapped by their thoughts. They are therefore unable to translate their thoughts into words.

Therefore, you should always concentrate on making statements, not asking questions. For instance, instead asking "Where did you buy the shirt?" You could say, "Your shirt looks nice and I'd like to purchase one." The child will be enticed to engage in conversation with you and let them to make comments on your assertion.

Wait patiently for the answer

Autism-related children can hear all you speak in clear and precise terms. But, it takes time for them to come up with a reaction. Most adults don't have time enough to see the response and ask a different question the child with autism. This causes disruptions in their brains and makes it difficult for them to answer any of these questions.

It can take around 20 to 30 seconds for a child of this age to get a response. It is important to allow the time and patience. Check how long your child is taking to reply. Keep the duration in mind for the next conversation.

Keep trying

There are two things that you must keep in mind. They are children and they are autistic. Both of these factors affect their reactions to social interactions and conversations. Therefore, you shouldn't expect to be successful after only a couple of trials. Continue to use your patience and kindness to reach out them.

There's a completely different world in the imagination of an autistic child. You shouldn't expect them to break out of it and be a part of the world of social interaction. The regular testing process will help you to understand the way they think and help you communicate your message simultaneously.

Create Routines Fun for Me

Early on in the spectrum of autism, you'll observe the love of predictable routine, ritual and routines in children.

Routines enable the child to discover a method of dealing with the various problems of their everyday life. But, certain rituals may become challenging to handle consistently. For example when your child prefers using the family toilet, it could be a problem when the child is old enough to be able to go to school. It is therefore essential that you learn to create and modify routines in accordance with the needs of the child.

What makes an autistic child need a regular routine?

Every individual is trying to control their surroundings to limit the possibility of unpredictability. But this practice is taken to a new level for children with ASD and autism. The fear of uncertainty causes them to be afraid of even the simplest things. The reason is that their brains try to overcome this fear by creating the most predictable routine for every possible scenario. However, the same routine can make the new experiences more terrifying for children.

A typical routine for children with autism typically involves food things, people, locations and ways of performing the task.

What are the reasons to focus on creating routines for your child?

Every day the autistic child battles with depression, anxiety, and a lack of certainty.

Routine is an instrument for the child to manage these problems. The ability to regulate and be predictable can bring peace to the child.

It's normal that you should be aware of the restrictions of routines that are part of the daily life for your children, particularly when your child won't let you to alter the routines. Yet, you should be a bit more inclined to create routines.

Why? !

Since, once you understand how to create an established routine, you'll also know how to alter your routine by switching it to another. In this way, you can give a sense stability to your child and offer health. This stability can be beneficial when you are trying to replace the ritual to an alternative.

How can you create fun routines?

The first step is in creating an effective routine. It is important to set up a variety of reminders during the first phases. It is possible to use visual aids to assist them in following an established routine every day. Try to make it as easy as possible, so the child is able to see and comprehend without assistance. The goal is to make each task enjoyable and familiar to the child.

When you have created a schedule, it is important to ensure the repeatability of the tasks is in the same way. But keep your expectations real. Don't try to force a routine upon the child.

Here are some activities that you can do to make your the routine enjoyable

Paint them

* Bring them to dance classes in special occasions.

* Host weekend parties at the house for your kids and other friends

* Play imitative

These are just a few examples of what you can do. But the most enjoyable job is to do something your child is excited about. Include some of them within different parts of a routine. This will help make schoolwork as well as other activities more exciting for the child.

Teachers who design routines for autistic children, they must be aware of two main elements:

* Keeping it entertaining and thrilling

Use routines to reach objectives in teaching

Teachers can select the right games and activities to increase the motor skills, social interaction and the language ability of autistic children.

How can we encourage the change between one practice to another?

Moving between activities, toys or routines require a consistent approach. The process is known as changing.

The initial step in preparing an adjustment in routine is to communicate. There are numerous methods to convey the possibility of a changes to children who have ASD.

Make use of visual elements

A list of notes or a collection of images as well as other visual elements can assist in explaining the shift. Start getting your child ready for school by showing them images of a school as well as other children as well as teachers. You can also use educational videos to help them comprehend the surroundings. It is also helpful when you plan to visit the city of your choice. Images of flights cities, locations in the city, and other locations will help your child prepare for these visual stimuli.

Let your child experience an unfamiliar place for a couple of times

When you are moving into the new house it is advisable to take your child for to the new place. Make sure they visit the new house frequently prior to eventually moving in. In the same way, you can request the school officials permission to meet with your child when the school day is over. The goal is to eliminate the fear of being in a new place from the area and ensure that your child is able to integrate into the new routines.

Rehearse your social interactions

Your child is fond of going to the same park each day. But , now that park is no longer open and you need to pick another one for your evening stroll. There are a variety of similar social events that require regular changes.

The best thing you could do is begin sharing stories of those experiences. Develop a sense that you are heroic in overcoming the challenges of changing routines. This can create an attitude of confidence and help prepare your child for the new social situations.

Be prepared with a plan "B"

Your plan could fail many times, so make sure you are well-prepared with a plan B always. This second option will be more secure. For instance, you could bring your favorite books, toys, or other things to soothe the child. Also, you can keep a distinct area in your mind that you can take your child to help calm him or her.

Reward and praise the person to those who try new routines.

Beginning a new routine can be an excellent thing for your child. It is important to encourage the feeling of accomplishment by giving praise and rewards. It is best to give them an item that is tangible and becomes the symbol of their achievement. The gift will help the child remember your satisfaction when he/she has finished a specific task. Thus, your child will be motivated to try the same thing over and over repeatedly. However, make sure to reinforce each attempt by giving a reward.

There is one thing you should be aware of that routines are a possibility in the event of autism. They can be effective as well as enjoyable and flexible while at the same time. From home to school , and any other public location routines can help your child to be happier at ease, calm, and secure.

I Love You No Whatever

If you have a child with autism caring for that child becomes your main concern. Medical facilities, treatments and therapies perform their job however it is essential for your child to feel loved.

There are two things you can do to ensure that you love your child who is autistic unconditionally. One is to let your child know that you cherish your child. The second is to look after yourself and remain positive throughout your life.

Check out the positive

Your enthusiasm is passed on to your child. Instead of thinking of autism as a disorder you should be more focused on the progress your child is showing. Be sure to show your appreciation with praise and reward. This will make your child feel loved and accepted.

It is essential to remain specific when praising the behavior. Your child should be aware of which behavior is appropriate and what isn't by you. Find innovative ways to show your happiness through reward and sweets. Allow extra time for play, or let them play with their toys or find other ways to convey a positive mindset to your child. So, you'll get regular progress from your child and you will be content too.

Show your love even if you don't think they'll

Following an aggressive breakdown or a mishap the child is scared. This is the crucial moment to be a loving parent and the teaching. This is not about enticing to encourage a negative behaviour. It is important to inform your child of the consequences of their actions. Also, make sure to tell them verbally that you will love your child regardless of the situation. This will help the child feel more comfortable and loved, which usually encourages positive behavior from these children.

Have fun with the child

Instead of doing a routine for obligation, get involved in games. Find fun and exciting tasks that you can work on with your child. Even if something seems silly or unimportant to you keep doing the task. Engage yourself to the child so that they feels connected to you. This helps open the door to autistic children if you've met him or them for the very first time.

Involve kids in your daily activities

The unpredictable nature of children could make you feel uncomfortable. It is crucial that you introduce them into your world in a secure way. A short excursion to the supermarket or to the bank or post office as well as other outings are crucial. You must take full charge of your child's fears But isolation is not the best solution. Let the child become accustomed with the world around them as well as feel appreciated.

Take some time to yourself

Mental health issues like depression stress, anxiety and damage to relationships are a possibility for caregivers. They can occur when you don't take good care of yourself and stress your mind with the obligation of taking care of others. Your mental and physical well-being can be affected by this way.

It is crucial to keep in mind that you are also a human. An ongoing effort to remain well-organized and ready will make you feel cut apart from the rest of the world. So, it's smart to make time to enjoy a positive attitude.

Set your child's schedule in line with your own in order that you are able to focus on self-care as well as the child's responsibilities. This will allow you to determine the causes of your anxiety. It is possible to create a plan to rid yourself of any negative emotions and love your child with all your heart.

Meditation is a great solution to your hyper-focused life. It allows your mind to relax and be conscious of your emotions and thoughts. You can speak to your own inner self and let go of the unnecessary worry and negative feelings.

An hour of exercise can revitalize your body and mind throughout the day. It is not necessary to schedule the gym into your busy schedule. Walk from the home to the store, or dance to your favourite music while cooking your food. If possible opt for yoga or any other exercise classes to connect with people your age and enjoy a relaxing time. It can replenish your mental and physical batteries.

Being able to manage daily tasks and caring for your child requires sound rest each night. Yoga, meditation, and relaxation can improve sleep quality. Thus, you'll begin taking more rest and will feel more confident.

The happiness and quality of your life will make your child feel valued and loved. The key is to find the right balance to keep your child, as well as you, happy. The time you spend with your friends wouldn't be a bad idea on a regular basis. It is possible to request a trustworthy teacher to watch your child while you spend time with your buddies. By knowing who you can assist, you to love your child more as an adult. Therefore, there's no reason not to spend time with hobbies as well as taking time to take care of yourself. Take a bath and dress in your most comfortable clothes, and then do your work as an adult.

Find the support you need to be helpful

You require all the help you can get from your friends and family members as well as experts. Involving yourself in counseling or support group can assist you to better understand the difficulties. You'll meet others parents or caregivers who are going through similar struggles. This will encourage you to cherish and help your child more. You will discover reliable sources and use those lessons to your daily life. This will allow you to take charge of your child more efficiently.

Do not let your love get in the form of treats

As parents, you cherish your child regardless of what. Sometimes, it's your love that prevents your child to receive proper treatment. If medical professionals suggest that you seek the assistance of experienced caregivers because of the severe ASD signs in the child it is your responsibility to listen. Your child's health is the first priority. Additionally, it can aid you in regaining your confidence and lead living a healthy life.

I'd Like To Be Loved Just Like Everyone else

In spite of all attention and concern an autistic child wants regular treatment from parents, teachers or caregivers as well as others. There are specific strategies to make the child be more at ease in their daily day life:

Do not talk as if your child isn't even in the same room.

Many people make the error of avoiding children when discussing their children. They assume that the lack of eye contact or silence indicates that the child is not paying attention to their words.

If parents discuss their issues with a child this could harm the child's mental state. A third party must not talk about autism whenever the child is in.

Ask a child who has ASD as a normal child. They will be able to answer your questions quickly. If you don't hear back do not be rude by discussing their state directly in front of them.

Accept the fact that their identity is not limited to autism.

Many professionals make the error of putting all the child's personality to be autism. It's a disorder that affects a large portion of a child's existence. But it's not his or her entire personality. There are certain desires and habits that a child develops through the help of his or her abilities. Recognizing the unique character of the child is important in making him feel valued. Don't connect all good and bad with autism. Do not say, "He is good at math due to autism." In the same way, a child may have a tendency to dislike himself despite having an autistic disorder.

Connecting all aspects of a child's personality to autism may cause them to lose their identity for the better. They must feel normal and have a sense self that is greater than the manifestation of a disorder. If you're in the presence of such children you have a responsibility to make sure that they feel comfortable with their own self-esteem. If a condition is associated with autism, you don't have to remind your child of that repeatedly.

Make sure to consider their viewpoint

It's not just about listening to what they have to say. It is important to listen and try to understand their point of view. People often overlook the majority of the words spoken by children with autism that makes them feel isolated and strange. Your patience can assist them to communicate their viewpoint regarding issues. Most of the time the views are valid and beneficial in helping the kids.

Do not let autism become an insufficiency

If people hear "autism," they think of it as a condition. This is the thought that hinders teachers, parents, and others to treat these children as normal.

The idea of treating autism as a condition is unproductive for parents. However, the issue becomes more serious when the child starts experiencing a sense of deficiency due to autism. The world around him is constantly pushing them to feel less and unimportant. This affects their self-esteem which is more serious than having autism.

Conclusion

It's surely been quite an experience to read this book. All this information can be quite a shock for anyone. Being aware that your child suffers from Autism is something most parents are never able to overcome. Although you are awed by your kid, it's hard to not wish that the world was different. However, they're not and you'll have to endure the situation.

Like we've discussed numerous times during this publication, you need to recognize the importance of your kid right now. You might have to care for him, but he's likely have to learn how to adapt, grow and flourish with the disorder. As we've seen in the previous chapter people suffering from ASD are able to live active and fulfilling lives, and you shouldn't need to worry about taking care of your child throughout his life. You'll get it eventually. Although it's a problem which the majority of people would like nothing to have to do with, it's certainly not an end in itself. In fact, it's actually a new beginning.

This book can serve as a reference those times when you are overwhelmed and confused about how to proceed in the care of your child. While it's not an actual book about parenting but it does provide valuable information about raising and interacting with your child. As you've learned that parenting isn't the most easy job you can do. Being a parent of an autistic child is even more difficult.

It all starts with knowing that, after all has been completed your child remains just a child. He is a child with mental and psychological developmental milestones he has to achieve, just like every other child. There are things he does that are hard to understand is a tantrum, avoids sharing, and throws temper tantrums. from sharing and puts everything in his mouth like any other child.

The only distinction could be that you child may be able to complete these milestones more slowly than other children. And this is where your care and love play a role. Your child will also require assistance in to interact with other children as the social skills he develops won't be as easy to master. You may need to employ methods like role-playing or explaining how to manage losing.

As we've outlined throughout the book, raising an autistic child is the same as parenting 2.0. You'll require all the knowledge you've learned from your children who are not autistic, and some fresh ones. The art of communicating with your children, organizing your schedule, and managing stress are at high on the list of things to do. Also, you'll need to know how to create a space that your child is able to flourish while finding innovative and practical solutions to every day issues.

www.ingramcontent.com/pod-product-compliance
Lightning Source LLC
Chambersburg PA
CBHW060326030426
42336CB00011B/1218